HUMAN ANATOMY AND PHYSIOLOGY

PATHOLOGY

NEW RESEARCH

HUMAN ANATOMY AND PHYSIOLOGY

Additional books in this series can be found on Nova's website under the Series tab.

Additional e-books in this series can be found on Nova's website under the E-book tab.

HUMAN ANATOMY AND PHYSIOLOGY

PATHOLOGY

NEW RESEARCH

JULIE M. VULTAGIONE
AND
KYLE N. FORESTER
EDITORS

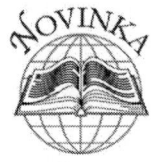

Nova Science Publishers, Inc.
New York

Copyright © 2012 by Nova Science Publishers, Inc.

All rights reserved. No part of this book may be reproduced, stored in a retrieval system or transmitted in any form or by any means: electronic, electrostatic, magnetic, tape, mechanical photocopying, recording or otherwise without the written permission of the Publisher.

For permission to use material from this book please contact us:
Telephone 631-231-7269; Fax 631-231-8175
Web Site: http://www.novapublishers.com

NOTICE TO THE READER

The Publisher has taken reasonable care in the preparation of this book, but makes no expressed or implied warranty of any kind and assumes no responsibility for any errors or omissions. No liability is assumed for incidental or consequential damages in connection with or arising out of information contained in this book. The Publisher shall not be liable for any special, consequential, or exemplary damages resulting, in whole or in part, from the readers' use of, or reliance upon, this material. Any parts of this book based on government reports are so indicated and copyright is claimed for those parts to the extent applicable to compilations of such works.

Independent verification should be sought for any data, advice or recommendations contained in this book. In addition, no responsibility is assumed by the publisher for any injury and/or damage to persons or property arising from any methods, products, instructions, ideas or otherwise contained in this publication.

This publication is designed to provide accurate and authoritative information with regard to the subject matter covered herein. It is sold with the clear understanding that the Publisher is not engaged in rendering legal or any other professional services. If legal or any other expert assistance is required, the services of a competent person should be sought. FROM A DECLARATION OF PARTICIPANTS JOINTLY ADOPTED BY A COMMITTEE OF THE AMERICAN BAR ASSOCIATION AND A COMMITTEE OF PUBLISHERS.

Additional color graphics may be available in the e-book version of this book.

Library of Congress Cataloging-in-Publication Data

Pathology : new research / editors, Julie M. Vultagione and Kyle N. Forester.
    p. ; cm.
Includes bibliographical references and index.
ISBN 978-1-62100-698-5 (softcover)
I. Vultagione, Julie M. II. Forester, Kyle N.
[DNLM: 1. Autopsy--methods. 2. Cause of Death. QZ 35]

616.07--dc23
                    2011037422

Published by Nova Science Publishers, Inc. † New York

Contents

Preface		vii
Chapter 1	Fatty Acid Oxidation Disorders on Sudden Unexpected Death in Infancy: Postmortem Screening with Metabolic Autopsy *Takuma Yamamoto, Hidekazu Tanaka, Yuko Emoto and Ryoji Matoba*	1
Chapter 2	Challenging the Authority of the Autopsy in Coronial Investigations *Belinda Carpenter, Gordon Tait, Michael Barnes and Charles Naylor*	35
Chapter 3	Psychopathology of Suicide in Bali *Toshiyuki Kurihara and Motoichiro Kato*	55
Chapter 4	Pathological Examination of Influenza Virus–Associated and Autoimmune Encephalitis/Encephalopathy in Children *Masaharu Hayashi, Yasuo Hachiya and Akihisa Okumura*	73
Chapter5	Histopathological Investigation in Forensic Autopsies *Tanuj Kanchan, Flora D. Lobo, Ritesh G. Menezes and B. Suresh Kumar Shetty*	91
Index		99

PREFACE

General pathology is a broad and complex scientific field which seeks to understand the mechanisms of injury to cells and tissues, as well as the body's means of responding to and repairing injury. Areas of study include cellular adaptation to injury, necrosis, inflammation, wound healing, and neoplasia. The foundation of pathology is the application of this knowledge to diagnose diseases in humans and animals. In this book, the authors present topical research in the study of pathology, including challenging the authority of the autopsy in coronial investigations; pathological examination of influenza virus-associated and autoimmune encephalitis/encephalopathy in children; histopathological investigation in forensic autopsies; psychopathology of suicide in Bali and the pathology of fatty acid oxidation disorders on sudden unexpected death in infancy

Chapter 1- In the field of forensic science the authors sometimes encounter an autopsy case of sudden infant death. The manner of death includes natural or external cause, except for unknown cases due to putrefaction or skeletonization. The common causes of sudden unexpected death in infancy are infection, cardiovascular anomaly, child abuse, metabolic disorders, and sudden infant death syndrome. Sudden infant death syndrome is defined as "the sudden death of an infant under one year of age, which remains unexplained after a thorough case investigation, including performance of a complete autopsy, examination of the death scene, and review of the clinical history". That is, sudden infant death syndrome is a natural disease that cannot be explained following a complete autopsy.

In the field of forensic science, at least in Japan, macroscopic examination, histopathological examination, and toxicological examination are routinely performed. Recently, autopsy imaging has been developed and is being performed in many institutions. Although morphological abnormalities can be detected during such examinations, they often fail to detect functional abnormalities. Molecular analyses or biochemical examinations are therefore needed.

In some institutions that have pediatric pathologists, sudden unexpected death in infancy cases caused by inherited metabolic disorders can be diagnosed by metabolic autopsy. However, autopsy cases of infants are not always performed by pediatric pathologists. Therefore, metabolic autopsy may not be classified as "a complete autopsy" during autopsy cases in the absence of a pediatric pathologist. Inherited metabolic disorders may, therefore, be underdiagnosed as a cause of sudden unexpected death in infancy or misdiagnosed as sudden infant death syndrome. In this chapter the authors focus on the importance of metabolic autopsy and also emphasize the necessity of expanded newborn screening.

The central purpose of this chapter is to address the tension between legal and medical discourses within the coronial/medico-legal system. In the context of a death investigation, medical expertise, manifest through the knowledge gained in an internal autopsy, is positioned as contributing the more valuable facts of the case, especially when contrasted with the evidence gathered at the scene of the death. The authors challenge this taken for granted understanding of medical knowledge in three ways: first, they examine the aspects of the history, philosophy and consequences of the processes by which the medical model gained its current dominance; second, they challenge the assumption that internal autopsy adds value to the death investigation, by utilising data from their own research in Australia; and finally, they engage with the debate about the purpose of a coronial/medico-legal investigation and role of an internal autopsy within that system.

Chapter 3- Although suicide is one of the major causes of death worldwide, research regarding suicide in developing countries is still lacking. In this chapter, the authors discuss the psychopathology of suicide in Bali, Indonesia. In the first section, they present research investigating the suicide rate in Bali. An examination of case records from police stations and interviews with police, community leaders, doctors, and victims' families was conducted. This investigation revealed that the annual suicide rate in Bali was 4.6 per 100,000 population in 2006. In the second section, they describe a psychological autopsy study comparing 60 suicide cases and 120 living controls matched for age, sex, and area of residence. This study identified the following risk factors for suicide: at least one diagnosis of an Axis-I mental disorder, low level of religious involvement, and severe interpersonal problems. Overall, 80.0% of the suicide cases were diagnosed with mental disorders; however, only 16.7% had visited a primary care health professional and none had received psychiatric treatment during the 1 month prior to death. These results highlight the importance of early recognition and treatment of mental disorders, religious activities, and interpersonal problem-solving strategies for suicide prevention in Bali.

Chapter 4- Despite advances in treatments with antibiotics and prophylaxis by vaccinations, influenza virus–associated encephalitis/encephalopathy tends to be intractable and may be a cause of mortality and severe sequelae in children. In order to clarify the pathogenesis of childhood-onset encephalitis/encephalopathy, the authors conducted pathological examinations of brain tissue sections of these patients. First, in this review, they summarize the neuropathological features of influenza virus–associated encephalitis/encephalopathy of patients in Japan and present data on the involvement of oxidative stress in acute necrotizing encephalopathy. Second, the authors review the significance of autoantibodies against the glutamate receptor, glutamic acid decarboxylase, and voltage-gated potassium channels in childhood-onset neurological disorders. Finally, the authors show their immunohistochemical data on antineuronal autoantibody screenings using patient sera on control brain sections. In Japan, the incidence of subacute and focal encephalitis/encephalopathy during which children repetitively develop episodes of psychological abnormalities, convulsions, and/or involuntary movements has increased. Immune-modulating treatments are effective, indicating the possible involvement of autoimmune mechanisms. The authors compared the immunehistochemical results using serum from patients in the acute disease phase with those using serum from patients in the convalescent phase and explored the presence or absence of immunoreactivity that was localized to the symptom-related brain area. In three-fifths of the subjects, symptom-related immunoreactivity was identified in the cerebral cortex, hippocampus, basal ganglia, and/or thalamus. This screening method was useful for investigating the pathogenesis of focal encephalitis/encephalopathy in children.

Chapter 5- Forensic autopsies are primarily conducted to determine the cause of death and to opine if the cause of death is in accordance with the postulated manner of death. These autopsies require photography, collection of evidentiary material and identification procedures, along with chemical analysis, histopathological evaluation, and other ancillary autopsy investigations. In cases of sudden unexpected deaths wherein even though the death may have occurred from an identifiable cause, the gross autopsy findings may be obscure or non-specific thus necessitating histopathological evaluation. Histopathological evaluation is however, not very commonly done in developing countries like India and its significance needs to be studied and emphasized in such countries. The present study was conducted in Kasturba Medical College, Mangalore, a medical institute affiliated to Manipal University in South India to highlight the importance of histopathological evaluation in medicolegal autopsies. Two hundred forensic autopsy cases were evaluated for histopathology in the associated Department of Pathology between January 2006 and September 2007. The autopsies were conducted by the Department of Forensic Medicine and the internal organs were subjected to histopathological evaluation in the Department of Pathology. Coronary atherosclerotic diseases, pneumonia and tuberculosis were the most frequent diagnoses observed in the autopsied cases. In the present case series, the authors have reviewed six of the unusual cases diagnosed solely by histopathological examination of the internal organs after autopsy during the aforementioned study period. The cases reviewed included a case of choriocarcinoma clinically diagnosed as septic abortion, acute leukemia manifesting as cerebral haemorrhage due to thrombocytopenia, tuberculous myocarditis presenting as sudden cardiac death, biliary cirrhosis in a chronic alcoholic, acute haemorrhagic pancreatitis as a cause of sudden death, and a case of sudden unexpected death due to malaria. The present research highlights on the decisive role of histopathological examination and the increasing trend of its usefulness in medicolegal work in recent times in developing countries like India.

In: Pathology: New Research
Editors: J. M. Vultagione et al.
ISBN: 978-1-62100-698-5
© 2012 Nova Science Publishers, Inc.

Chapter 1

FATTY ACID OXIDATION DISORDERS ON SUDDEN UNEXPECTED DEATH IN INFANCY: POSTMORTEM SCREENING WITH METABOLIC AUTOPSY

Takuma Yamamoto[a], Hidekazu Tanaka[b], Yuko Emoto[a] and Ryoji Matoba[a]

[a] Department of Legal Medicine, Osaka University Graduate School of Medicine, Japan
[b] Department of Pharmacology, Osaka University Graduate School of Medicine, Osaka, Japan

ABSTRACT

In the field of forensic science we sometimes encounter an autopsy case of sudden infant death. The manner of death includes natural or external cause, except for unknown cases due to putrefaction or skeletonization. The common causes of sudden unexpected death in infancy are infection, cardiovascular anomaly, child abuse, metabolic disorders, and sudden infant death syndrome. Sudden infant death syndrome is defined as "the sudden death of an infant under one year of age, which remains unexplained after a thorough case investigation, including performance of a complete autopsy, examination of the death scene, and review of the clinical history". That is, sudden infant death syndrome is a natural disease that cannot be explained following a complete autopsy.

In the field of forensic science, at least in Japan, macroscopic examination, histopathological examination, and toxicological examination are routinely performed. Recently, autopsy imaging has been developed and is being performed in many institutions. Although morphological abnormalities can be detected during such examinations, they often fail to detect functional abnormalities. Molecular analyses or biochemical examinations are therefore needed.

In some institutions that have pediatric pathologists, sudden unexpected death in infancy cases caused by inherited metabolic disorders can be diagnosed by metabolic autopsy. However, autopsy cases of infants are not always performed by pediatric pathologists. Therefore, metabolic autopsy may not be classified as "a complete autopsy" during autopsy cases in the absence of a pediatric pathologist. Inherited metabolic disorders may, therefore, be underdiagnosed as a cause of sudden unexpected death in infancy or misdiagnosed as sudden infant death syndrome. In this chapter we focus on the importance of metabolic autopsy and also emphasize the necessity of expanded newborn screening.

1. INTRODUCTION

Forensic pathologists keep in mind the story of "Scientific sleuths solve a murder mystery" [1]. In this story, a mother, whose son died suddenly after having labored breathing, uncontrollable vomiting, and gastric distress, was sentenced to life in prison as a murder to her son, because the son was diagnosed as ethylene glycol poisoning. However, the diagnosis was later corrected to methylmalonic acidemia by "metabolic autopsy" [2].

In the field of forensic science we sometimes encounter an autopsy case of sudden infant death. Pathologists use diverse terminologies for the classification of sudden infant deaths, including "unascertained", "sudden unexplained death in infancy", "sudden unexpected death in infancy" (SUDI), and "sudden infant death syndrome" (SIDS) [3,4]. In this chapter we define SUDI as sudden unexpected death occurring before 12 months of age. If the cause of SUDI remains unexplained after a case investigation, it is termed as SIDS [5].

The manner of death includes natural or external cause, except for unknown cases due to putrefaction or skeletonization. The common causes of SUDI are infection, cardiovascular anomaly, child abuse, metabolic disorders

[6-8], and SIDS. Despite declines in SIDS rates following risk reduction campaigns, SIDS continues to be the leading cause of death for infants between 1 month and 1 year of age in developed countries [9]. SIDS is defined as "the sudden death of an infant under one year of age, which remains unexplained after a thorough case investigation, including performance of a complete autopsy, examination of the death scene, and review of the clinical history" [10]. That is, SIDS is a natural disease that cannot be explained following a complete autopsy.

In the field of forensic science, at least in Japan, macroscopic examination, histopathological examination, and toxicological examination are routinely performed. Recently, autopsy imaging has been developed and is being performed in many institutions. Although morphological abnormalities can be detected during such examinations, they often fail to detect functional abnormalities. Molecular analyses or biochemical examinations are therefore needed.

Congenital cardiovascular defects and serious infection can be detected by conventional autopsy with macroscopic or histopathological examination. However, some diseases such as potential inherited metabolic disorders (IMDs) are more difficult to diagnose at autopsy than cardiovascular defects or serious infection. In some institutions that have pediatric pathologists, SUDI cases caused by IMDs can be diagnosed by metabolic autopsy (Table 1) [5,11-15]. However, autopsy cases of infants are not always performed by pediatric pathologists. Therefore, metabolic autopsy may not be classified as "a complete autopsy" during autopsy cases in the absence of a pediatric pathologist [11]. IMDs may, therefore, be underdiagnosed as a cause of SUDI or misdiagnosed as SIDS [6,7,16]. In this chapter we focus on the importance of metabolic autopsy and also emphasize the necessity of expanded newborn screening (NBS).

Table 1. Proportion of inherited metabolic disorders among sudden unexpected death in infancy

Reference	No. of cases	No. positive
Bennett et al. (1994) [11]	58	6 (10.3%)
Lundemose et al. (1997) [12]	79	3 (3.8%)
Boles et al. (1998) [13]	418	14 (3.3%)
Rinaldo et al. (1999) [14]	>500	63
Chace et al. (2001) [15]	7058	66 (0.93%)
Wilcox et al. (2002) [5]	247	3 (1.2%)

2. MECHANISMS OF FATTY ACID OXIDATION

The physiological response during fasting is the utilization of stored hepatic and muscle glycogen to maintain normoglycemia. However, when glycogen reserves are depleted, lipid stores are the main source of energy supply. Triglycerides are degraded to fatty acids by lipolysis and fatty acids are utilized for energy supply. Mitochondrial fatty acid oxidation is therefore essential for energy production during fasting, febrile illness, or increased muscular activity. In newborns especially, energy production depends heavily on fatty acids as they have limited glycogen reserves. Mitochondrial fatty acid oxidation also synthesizes ketone bodies, which are utilized as an alternative energy source in brain [17].

Several types of fatty acid oxidation processes are known in the cell: alpha-, beta-, and omega-oxidation. These processes take place in mitochondria or peroxisomes. The most common pathway is beta-oxidation in the mitochondrial matrix, which is responsible for the degradation of straight-chain fatty acids [18].

2.1. Plasma Membrane Fatty Acid Transport

Fatty acids with carbon chain-lengths of primarily 18 carbons or less are metabolized in mitochondria, while very long-chain fatty acids, longer than 20 carbons, are metabolized by peroxisomal beta-oxidation.

Whereas medium- and short-chain fatty acids can passively enter into the mitochondrial matrix, the transportation of long-chain fatty acid (LCFA) is dependent on the carnitine shuttle. LCFA is transported into cytosol by means of plasma membrane LCFA transporters (FATP; with six different types, designated FATP1 to 6) and fatty acid translocase (FAT). LCFA is then activated to acyl-CoA ester by ATP-dependent acyl-CoA synthetase (ACS) located at the plasma membrane, whereas medium- and short-chain fatty acids are activated within the mitochondrial matrix [19].

2.2. Mitochondrial Transport of Fatty Acids

Carnitine is also transported into cytosol by means of plasma membrane organic cation/carnitine transporter 2 (OCTN2 transporter, also called carnitine transporter). Carnitine palmitoyl transferase I (CPT I), which is situated on the outer mitochondrial membrane (OMM), forms long-chain acyl-carnitine from acyl-CoA and free carnitine. The long-chain acyl-carnitine is transported into the mitochondrial matrix by means of carnitine-acylcarnitine translocase (CACT). Carnitine palmitoyl transferase II (CPT II), which is situated on the inner aspect of the inner mitochondrial membrane (IMM), converts long-chain acylcarnitine to long-chain acyl-CoA. The released carnitine is recycled for subsequent reutilization via CACT [17].

Malonyl-CoA inhibits CPT I activity and prevents formation of long-chain acyl-carnitine in a postprandial state. During fasting, on the contrary, when the level of malonyl-CoA decreases, CPT I activity increases and more long-chain acyl-carnitines are formed [17].

2.3. Fatty Acid Beta-oxidation

Beta-oxidation represents a spiral pathway that includes four repetitive enzymatic reactions that result in the removal of two-carbon-unit acetyl-CoA. The first step is an FAD-dependent acyl-CoA dehydrogenase reaction by very-long-chain acyl-CoA dehydrogenase (VLCAD), medium-chain acyl-CoA dehydrogenase (MCAD), and short-chain acyl-CoA dehydrogenase (SCAD). This leads to the formation of 2-enoyl-CoA. Although long-chain acyl-CoA dehydrogenase (LCAD) has substrate chain-length specificity between VLCAD and MCAD, no human case of LCAD deficiency has been described. Acyl-CoA dehydrogenase 9 (ACAD9), which is another acyl-CoA dehydrogenase, also acts on long-chain substrates. The second step involves hydration of the double bond to produce 3-hydroxyacyl-CoA with 2-enoyl-CoA hydratase. The third step involves NAD-dependent dehydrogenation at the 3-hydroxy position to yield 3-ketoacyl-CoA species with long-chain 3-hydroxyacyl-CoA dehydrogenase (LCHAD) and 3-hydroxyacyl-CoA dehydrogenase (HAD). The last step involves thiolytic cleavage of 3-ketoacyl-CoA to yield acetyl-CoA and two-carbon chain-shortened acyl-CoA. The enzymes responsible for this reaction are long-chain 3-ketoacyl-CoA thiolase (LCKAT), medium-chain 3-ketoacyl-CoA thiolase (MCKAT), and short-chain 3-ketoacyl-CoA thiolase (SCKAT) [18,20]. SCKAT is also known as beta-ketothiolase (beta-KT) and represents a common step with the metabolism of isoleucine. Beta-KT deficiency is therefore categorized as organic acid disorder [17].

Acetyl-CoA is finally fully degraded to CO_2 and H_2O via the Krebs cycle. The electrons generated by FAD-dependent dehydrogenation are transferred via electron transfer flavoprotein (ETF) and ETF dehydrogenase (ETFDH) to ubiquinone, which are then passed to the respiratory chain complex, together with electrons from NAD-dependent dehydrogenation.

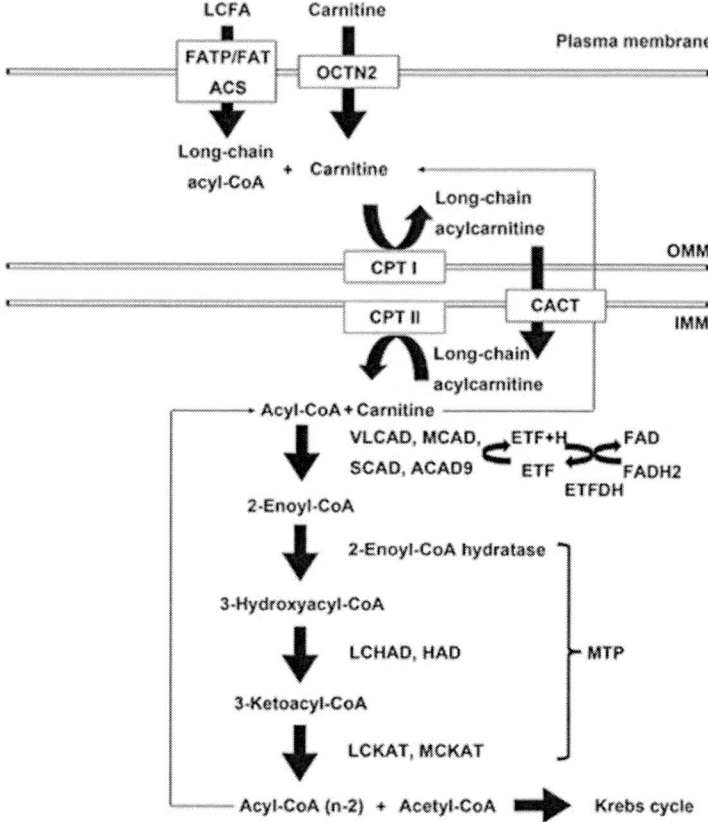

Figure 1. Fatty acid oxidation pathway. *Abbreviations:* ACAD9, acyl-CoA dehydrogenase 9; ACS, acyl-CoA synthetase; CACT, carnitine-acylcarnitine translocase; CPT, carnitine palmitoyl transferase; ETF, electron transfer flavoprotein; ETFDH, ETF dehydrogenase; FAT, fatty acid tranlocase; FATP, fatty acid transporter; HAD, 3-hydroxyacyl-CoA dehydrogenase; IMM, inner mitochondrial membrane; LCFA, long-chain fatty acid; LCHAD, long-chain 3-hydroxyacyl-CoA dehydrogenase; LCKAT, long-chain 3-ketoacyl-CoA thiolase; MCAD, medium-chain acyl-CoA dehydrogenase; MCKAT, medium-chain 3-ketoacyl-CoA thiolase; MTP, mitochondrial trifunctional protein; OCTN2, organic cation/carnitine transporter 2; OMM, outer mitochondrial membrane; SCAD, short-chain acyl-CoA dehydrogenase; VLCAD, very-long-chain acyl-CoA dehydrogenase.

The metabolism of unsaturated fatty acids with cis double bonds requires auxiliary enzymes in addition to the enzymes necessary for saturated fatty acid metabolism. 2,4-Dienoyl-CoA reductase is involved in the metabolism of all unsaturated fatty acids with double bonds at even-numbered positions and some unsaturated fatty acids with double bonds at odd-numbered positions [21].

The oxidation pathway is summarized in Figure 1. Enzymes for long-chain acyl-CoA, such as VLCAD and LCHAD, are located on the inner mitochondrial membrane, while enzymes for medium- or short-chain acyl-CoA, such as MCAD, SCAD, and short-chain enoyl-CoA hydratase, are present in the mitochondrial matrix [18]. Therefore, long-chain acyl-CoA is catalyzed on the inner mitochondrial membrane, while medium- and short-chain acyl-CoA are catalyzed in the mitochondrial matrix.

3. FATTY ACID OXIDATION DISORDERS

Since the first report of fatty acid oxidation disorder (FAOD) in 1973 as CPT II deficiency in an adult with rhabdomyolysis and myoglobinuria [22], many FAODs have been reported. Energetic deficiency of heart may be associated with cardiomyopathy and cardiac arrhythmia, while the accumulation of fatty acids in liver and muscles can cause fatty liver, hepatomegaly, muscle weakness, or hypotonia [18].

3.1. Primary Carnitine Deficiency

Primary carnitine deficiency (OMIM 212140) is caused by mutation in the *SLC22A5* gene (OMIM 603377), which is located on 5q31.1. The gene encodes a 63-kDa polypeptide.

Primary carnitine deficiency is caused by a lack of functional OCTN2 transporter. It has a frequency of about 1:40,000 newborns in Japan [23]. In infancy, it is often encountered before 2 years of age, with symptoms including decreased feeding, irritability, lethargy, and decreased responsiveness. Hepatomegaly is a frequent presentation. In older children, cardiomyopathy and muscle weakness are often presenting symptoms. Untreated patients can develop coma and sudden death [24]. A few patients live completely asymptomatically and are not diagnosed until their child is affected [25].

3.2. CPT I Deficiency

CPT I has three different isoforms. It is the only fatty acid oxidation enzyme to exist in tissue-specific isoforms. They are encoded by different genes: liver-type (encoded by the *CPT1A* gene located on 11q13), muscle-type (encoded by the *CPT1B* gene located on 22q13), and brain-type (encoded by the *CPT1C* gene located on 19q13) [24,26]. The *CPT1A* gene (OMIM 600528) encodes an 88-kDa polypeptide.

Liver-type CPT I deficiency (OMIM 255120) was first described in 1981 in an 8-month-old infant patient with fasting-induced non-ketotic hypoglycemia [27]. The first presenting symptom is Reye-like syndrome with hypoketotic hypoglycemia and hepatomegaly. Some patients present heart involvement, which is classically absent in CPT I deficiency [26].

3.3. CPT II Deficiency

CPT II deficiency was first described in 1973 [22]. It is now categorized into three forms: neonatal (OMIM 608836) [28-30], infantile (OMIM 600649) [31], and adult (OMIM 255110) [22]. The infantile form usually manifests between 6 and 24 months of age. It shows recurrent attacks of hypoketotic hypoglycemia resulting in coma and seizures, liver failure, and transient hepatomegaly. About one half of cases have heart involvement with cardiomyopathy and arrhythmia, and some cases result in SUDI. The neonatal form is more severe than the infantile form. Many sudden death cases are reported, most often during the first month of life. The adult form often manifests between 6 and 20 years of age, and is characterized by recurrent attacks of myalgia and muscle stiffness with myoglobinuria [24,26,32,33].

3.4. CACT Deficiency

CACT deficiency (OMIM 212138) is caused by mutation in the *SLC25A20* gene (OMIM 613698), which is located on 3p21.31. The gene encodes a 33-kDa polypeptide.

CACT deficiency was first described in 1992 by Stanley et al. in a 36-hour-old neonate [34]. It occurs in the neonatal period and in infants up to 15 months of age. The severe neonatal form presents with cardiomyopathy and multiple organ involvement. Most reported patients became symptomatic in the neonatal period with a rapidly progressive deterioration and a high mortality rate. The milder hypoglycemic form presents with normal growth, except for hypoglycemia [35].

3.5. VLCAD Deficiency

VLCAD deficiency (OMIM 201475) was first described in 1993 [36-38]. VLCAD deficiency is categorized into three forms: the severe childhood, the milder childhood, and the adult forms. The severe childhood form usually occurs in the neonatal period and has a high mortality rate. Cardiomyopathy, hepatomegaly, and hypotonia are frequently observed. The milder childhood form is characterized by delayed onset. The main clinical feature at presentation is hypoketotic hypoglycemia, hepatomegaly without cardiomyopathy, and hypotonia. The adult form is characterized by muscle pain, rhabdomyolysis, and myoglobinuria [39].

Patients who had been reported as having LCAD deficiency were subsequently shown to have VLCAD deficiency [38,40,41]. No confirmed human case of LCAD deficiency has therefore been described to date.

3.6. LCHAD, MTP, and LCKAT Deficiencies

Mitochondrial trifunctional protein (MTP, also called TFP) complex contains three enzyme activities: long-chain 2-enoyl-CoA hydratase (LCEH), LCHAD, and LCKAT [42,43]. The first two enzymes reside on the alpha subunit of the MTP complex, whereas LCKAT resides on the beta subunit.

Diseases of the MTP complex comprise two categories: isolated LCHAD deficiency (OMIM 609016) and general MTP deficiency (OMIM 609015). LCHAD deficiency is defined by the sole reduction of LCHAD activity, while MTP deficiency is defined by reduced activity of all three MTP enzymes. Recently, in 2006, Das et al. reported a case of LCKAT deficiency resulting from mutations in the *HADHB* gene, with death at 6 weeks of age resulting from pulmonary edema and cardiomyopathy [44].

The clinical manifestation of LCHAD and MTP deficiencies cannot be distinguished, and acylcarnitine analysis shows the same biochemical profile. Wanders et al. described a child with sudden infant death and accumulation of long-chain 3-hydroxy-fatty acids in 1989 [45,46]. Three years after that, MTP deficiency was first described in 1992 [47,48]. LCHAD and MTP deficiencies are categorized into three forms: a lethal cardiomyopathic form, an infant-onset hepatic form, and a late-onset neuromyopathic form. LCHAD and MTP deficiencies in infancy and early childhood present as fasting hypoketotic hypoglycemia, hepatomegaly, hepatoencephalopathy, hypotonia, areflexia, rhabdomyolysis, and cardiomyopathy, leading to sudden death. The late-onset neuromyopathic form is characterized by long-term complications such as retinopathy and peripheral neuropathy, which are not seen in any other FAODs [49, 50].

3.7. MCAD Deficiency

MCAD deficiency (OMIM 201450) was first described in 1976 [51]. MCAD deficiency is the most common FAOD in the world. The global frequency is 1:10,000-27,000, but is 1:50,000 in Japan [52]. MCAD deficiency usually first presents between a few months and 3 years of age, although neonatal and adult onset type have also been described. Symptoms include hypoketotic hypoglycemia, hypotonia, lethargy, and vomiting, leading to encephalopathy, coma, and sudden death [53].

MCAD deficiency is the first definite diagnosis of IMDs in an infant who was initially considered to be SIDS [54, 55]. An 18-month-old infant with non-specific malaise and mild infection of the upper respiratory tract suffered a grand mal convulsion and died suddenly. Autopsy showed diffuse fatty changes to viscera and he was eventually shown to have had MCAD deficiency.

3.8. MCKAT Deficiency

Only one case with MCKAT deficiency (OMIM 602199) has been reported to date [56]. A Japanese male neonate died at 13 days of age after presenting at 2 days of age with vomiting, dehydration, metabolic acidosis, liver dysfunction, and terminal rhabdomyolysis with myoglobinuria. A systematic study of the catalytic activities of beta-oxidation enzymes revealed a deficiency of MCKAT.

3.9. HAD Deficiency

HAD deficiency (OMIM 231530) is caused by mutation in the *HADH* gene (OMIM 601609), which is located on 4q22-q26. The gene encodes a 33-kDa polypeptide. The HAD enzyme has a broad chain-length specificity from medium- to short-chain.

The first patient with HAD deficiency was reported in 1991 by Tein et al. in a 16-year-old girl, resulting in juvenile-onset recurrent myoglobinuria, hypoketotic hypoglycemic encephalopathy, and hypertrophic/dilated cardiomyopathy [57], although it was initially considered as a short-chain 3-hydroxyacyl-CoA dehydrogenase deficiency [58]. HAD deficiency presents with fasting-induced vomiting, ketosis, hypoglycemia, hepatoencephalopathy, myopathy, and cardiomyopathy, which are often seen in other FAODs. The important feature of HAD deficiency is hyperinsulinism [59].

3.10. SCAD Deficiency

Turnbull et al. reported the case of a 53-year-old woman who presented with a lipid-storage myopathy and low concentrations of carnitine in skeletal muscle in 1984 [60]. However, later in 1995, this patient was proposed as not having had primary SCAD deficiency [61]. Amendt et al. described the first patient with SCAD deficiency (OMIM 201470) in 1987 [62]. Clinical symptoms in SCAD deficiency appear early in life, generally under 5 years of age, and include developmental delay, behavioral disorders, epilepsy, hypotonia, and hypoglycemia [63]. Most patients have not presented with the classic signs of hypoketotic hypoglycemia, recurrent rhabdomyolysis, or cardiomyopathy, which are often seen in other FAODs. The reason is that, since SCAD is only needed at the end of beta-oxidation cycle, the fatty acid oxidation pathway function preceding it may be sufficient for neoglucogenesis and ketogenic capability. MCAD may also partially compensate for SCAD enzyme deficiency because of an overlap of substrate specificity [64].

3.11. ACAD9 Deficiency

ACAD9 is one of the acyl-CoA dehydrogenases, which was first described in 2002 [65]. ACAD9 deficiency (OMIM 61112) was first described in 2007 in three patients who presented sudden death with Reye-like syndrome, recurrent episodes of acute liver dysfunction, and cardiomyopathy resulting in death, respectively [66].

3.12. Multiple acyl-CoA Dehydrogenase dEficiency

Multiple acyl-CoA dehydrogenation deficiency (MADD) (OMIM 231680), also called glutaric aciduria type II, is due to a defect in either the alpha or beta subunit of ETF (ETFA; OMIM 608053, ETFB; OMIM 130410) or ETFDH (OMIM 231675). These enzymes transfer electrons from mitochondrial FAD-dependent dehydrogenases to the respiratory chain complex.

It is divided into three clinical forms: a neonatal-onset form with congenital anomalies (type I), a neonatal-onset form without congenital anomalies (type II), and a late-onset form (type III). The neonatal-onset forms are usually fatal and present severe non-ketotic hypoglycemia, metabolic acidosis, and excretion of large amounts of metabolites [67].

3.13. 2,4-Dienoyl-CoA Reductase Deficiency

The first patient with 2,4-dienoyl-CoA reductase deficiency (OMIM 222745) was described in 1990 [68] and is the only patient reported so far. The patient was a black female, presenting in the neonatal period with persistent hypotonia. Biochemical studies revealed hyperlysinemia, hypocarnitinemia, a normal organic acid profile, and an unusual acylcarnitine species in both urine and blood. The new metabolite was positively identified as 2-trans,4-cis-decadienoylcarnitine, derived from incomplete oxidation of linoleic acid. In spite of dietary therapy, the patient died from respiratory acidosis at 4 months of age.

4. POSTMORTEM DIAGNOSIS

Clinical features in FAODs are shown in Table 2 [17, 18, 69]. However, routine postmortem investigation can detect only a small proportion of these features: Reye-like syndrome, cardiomyopathy, or rhabdomyolysis. Clinical symptoms are often unknown in sudden death and biochemical laboratory data are unreliable because of postmortem changes.

Table 2. Clinical features in fatty acid oxidation disorders

Reye-like syndrome
Cyclic vomiting syndrome
Hypotonia or myopathy
Peripheral neuropathy
Loss of consciousness
Sudden death
Hypoketotic or ketotic hypoglycemia
Cardiomyopathy, Cardiac arrhythmia
Metabolic acidosis
AFLP/HELLP
Recurrent rhabdomyolysis
Dicarboxylic aciduria
Carnitine deficiency
Fulminant liver disease

Abbreviations: AFLP, acute fatty liver of pregnancy; HELLP, hypertension, elevated liver enzymes, and low platelets.

4.1. Histopathological Examination

Reye's syndrome is characterized by hepatic steatosis [70] and it is well known that FAODs manifest as Reye-like syndrome [71]. In infants, vacuolization of hepatocytes is often shown because of the presence of glycogen granules, for which hematoxylin and eosin staining alone is sometimes inadequate. To detect hepatic steatosis, Sudan III or Oil Red O staining are recommended. According to previous SUDI reports, about 5% of SUDI cases had hepatic steatosis (Table 3) [13,14,55,72-74]. In the Japanese population, 13.5% had hepatic steatosis [73]. Fat staining should be performed routinely in autopsy cases of infants.

4.2. Acylcarnitine Analysis

One of the first acylcarnitine identifications was described in 1977 with gas chromatography/mass spectrometry [75] and one of the earliest clinical applications of liquid chromatography/mass spectrometry for acylcarnitine analysis was reported in 1983 [76]. Improvements in the analysis of acylcarnitines and clinical diagnosis of FAODs occurred with tandem mass spectrometry (MS/MS) [77]. In 2001, Chace et al. reported a large series of postmortem acylcarnitine analysis using MS/MS [15], while many studies and case reports on postmortem samples were reported prior to 2001 [11-14,78-82]. The utility of postmortem metabolic screening with MS/MS has been subsequently reported [5].

Table 3. Relationship between fatty liver and sudden unexpected death in infancy

Reference	No. of cases	No. positive
Sinclair-Smith et al. (1976) [72]	200	10 (5.0%)
Howat et al. (1985) [55]	200	14 (7.0%)
Boles et al. (1998) [13]	418	37 (8.9%)
Sawaguchi et al. (1998) [73]	89	12 (13.5%)
Rinaldo et al. (1999) [14]	>500	51
Yang et al. (2007) [74]	220	16 (7.3%)

About 5-10% of SUDI cases could be diagnosed as FAODs by postmortem acylcarnitine analysis. However, some authors have reported an infrequent relationship between SUDI and FAODs [83-86], although this has been debated [79]. First, these reports did not focus on all FAODs, as the mutational analysis included only common mutations or the most common FAODs. Second, the criteria for SUDI were confusing. For example, some authors excluded cases with hepatic steatosis from SUDI groups.

Applying the data from newborn screening or high-risk selective screening to postmortem interpretation would produce a false-positive risk. Because MS/MS profiles from postmortem blood samples are characterized by increases in free carnitine and short-chain acylcarnitines [15], it is difficult to distinguish between postmortem changes and the diseases in which free carnitine increases, such as CPT I deficiency. Indeed, determination of the C0/(C16+C18) ratio in CPT I deficiency is recommended for newborn screening [87]; however, the ratio increases in almost all postmortem samples [88]. The estimation of short-chain acylcarnitines in postmortem samples is a challenge for the future.

In MCAD deficiency, medium-chain acylcarnitines such as C6, C8, C10, and C10:1 are increased. The ratio of C8 to C10 is available for differentiating MCAD deficiency from other FAODs. In VLCAD deficiency, long-chain acylcarnitines such as C14:1, C14, C16:1, C16, C18:1, and C18 are increased. The ratio of C14:1 to C12:1 is available for differentiating VLCAD deficiency from other LCFA disorders. In CPT II and CACT deficiencies, very long-chain acylcarnitines such as C16, C18, and C18:1 are increased. The ratio of C16 to C14:1 is available for differentiating CPT II and CACT deficiencies from other FAODs. In LCHAD and MTP deficiencies, long-chain hydroxyacylcarnitines such as C16OH, C18:1OH, and C18OH are increased. The ratio of C16OH to C16 is available for differentiating LCHAD and MTP deficiencies from other FAODs. In MADD, the ratio of long- to medium-chain multiple acylcarnitines is increased to mild-to-moderate extent. Such profiles are also seen in non-pathological samples, so the diagnosis of MADD is consequently challenging. In primary carnitine deficiency, free carnitine and acylcarnitines are decreased. As similarly low levels are often seen in insufficient or poor blood specimens, it should be confirmed whether the amino acid profile is consistently increased in autopsy blood specimens [15].

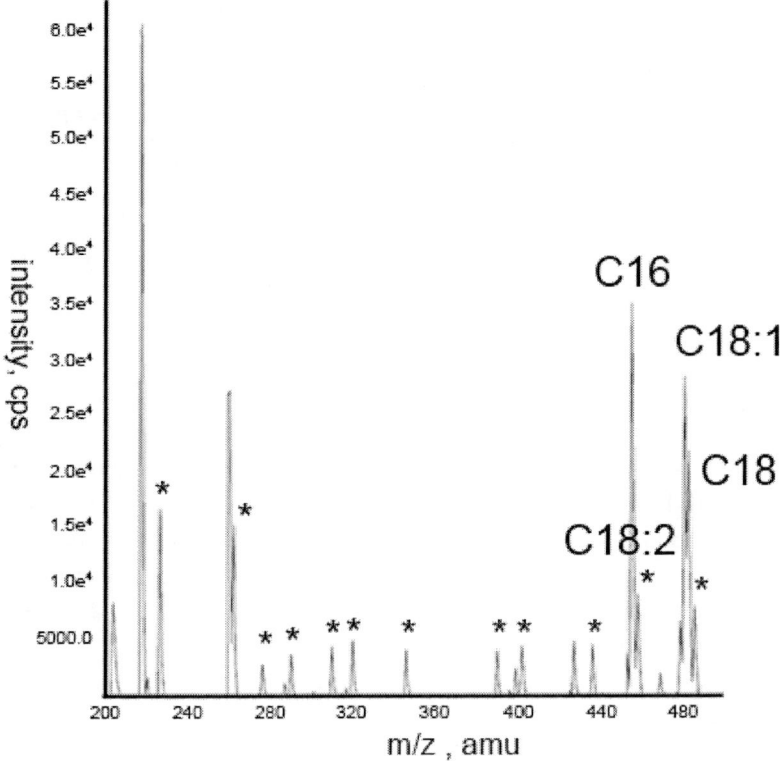

* Internal standard.

Figure 2. The acylcarnitine profile of the postmortem blood spot from an infant who died by CPT II deficiency.

The acylcarnitine profile of the postmortem blood spot from an infant who died by CPT II deficiency is shown in Figure 2. The infant died at 6 months of age after mild upper respiratory infection. The acylcarnitine profile of CPT II deficiency is the same as that of CACT deficiency. Therefore, it is impossible to distinguish between CPT II and CACT deficiencies by acylcarnitine analysis. In this case, mutational analysis revealed that the infant had a compound heterozygote in the *CPT2* gene [88].

It would be better to perform determination using the NBS Guthrie card if it is available and stored frozen, because postmortem changes make it difficult to interpret postmortem acylcarnitine profiles [88,89]. Rashed et al. reported postmortem acylcarnitine analysis in bile with two cases of LCHAD deficiency and one case of glutaryl-CoA dehydrogenase deficiency, thus demonstrating the benefit of acylcarnitine analysis in bile [80]. One characteristic of acylcarnitine profiles with postmortem bile includes high levels of long- and medium-chain acylcarnitines, i.e., C10:1, C10, C12:1, C12, C14:1, and C14, and relatively low levels of short-chain acylcarnitines. Another characteristic is the increase in the peak at m/z 342. This peak may be produced by a component in bile, although it would be suggestive of C8:1 [15].

Acylcarnitine analysis does not burden a conventional autopsy, because some toxicological screening can be achieved from the same postmortem blood specimen used for metabolic screening [15].

4.3. Mutational Analysis

One method for making a definite diagnosis is DNA analysis. Many FAODs are inherited in an autosomal recessive manner. Homozygous mutations or compound heterozygous mutations are reported to cause each disorder. The complete cDNA sequencing and the complete genomic sequencing of exons with each flanking intronic regions are recommended. Screening for the more common mutations is also performed for some FAODs; CPT II, LCHAD, MTP, and MCAD deficiencies have common disease-causing mutations.

4.3.1. CPT II Deficiency

CPT II deficiency is encoded by the *CPT2* gene (OMIM 600650), which spans 20 kb and contains 5 exons. The gene is located on chromosome 1p32.

In CPT II deficiency, more than 70 mutations have been reported, among which some common mutations exist. They are divided into severe (e.g., R151Q, P227L, D328G, R382K, F383Y) and mild (e.g., P50H, S113L, R161W) mutations [26]. At least three polymorphisms (F352C, V368I, and M647V) are also detected. Whereas these polymorphisms do not effect enzymatic activities [90, 91], they are associated with influenza-associated encephalopathy [92, 93]. It remains controversial whether these polymorphisms are related to clinical symptoms. Non-exonic region substitutions are also detected, which affect splicing. This splicing site substitution causes exon skip, leading an unstable mRNA or a premature stop codon [94, 95].

4.3.2. VLCAD Deficiency

VLCAD deficiency is encoded by the *ACADVL* gene (OMIM 609575), which spans 5.4 kb and contains 20 exons. The gene is located on chromosome 17p13.

Many different mutations have been detected in almost all exons [39], although no prevalent mutation has been detected [96]. Common polymorphisms are G43D and P266A [97].

4.3.3. LCHAD and MTP Deficiencies

The alpha subunit of MTP is encoded by the *HADHA* gene (OMIM 600890) and the beta subunit by the *HADHB* gene (OMIM 143450). They are composed of 20 and 16 exons, respectively. Both genes are located on chromosome 2p23.

LCHAD deficiency is caused by mutations of the alpha subunit. It results in reduced LCHAD activity, while LCEH and LCKAT activities remain normal. In contrast, MTP deficiency is caused by various mutations in either the alpha or beta subunit, which results in reduced activities for all three enzymes. The reason why the alpha-subunit mutations cause MTP deficiency is that these mutations disturb the whole complex and result in degradation of the protein [49, 98, 99].

The most common mutation is G1528C (E474Q) in exon 15 of the alpha subunit [100]. It has also been reported that an intronic exonization can be caused by a deep intronic mutation and result in MTP deficiency [101].

4.3.4. MCAD Deficiency

MCAD deficiency is encoded by the *ACADM* gene (OMIM 607008), which spans 44 kb and contains 12 exons. The gene is located on chromosome 1p31.

Many different mutations have been detected in almost all exons [96]. The most common mutation of MCAD deficiency is A985G (K304E).

4.3.5. SCAD Deficiency

SCAD deficiency is encoded by the *ACADS* gene (OMIM 606885), which spans 13 kb and contains 10 exons. The gene is located on chromosome 12q22.

More than 35 inactivating mutations and two polymorphisms have been reported. The C511T (R147W) and G625A (G185S) substitutions are relatively common in the general population [64], whereas Gregersen et al. demonstrated that homozygosity for one of the polymorphisms is associated with an increased incidence of elevated ethylmalonic acid excretion [102].

4.4. Enzymatic Analysis

Another method for making a definite diagnosis is enzymatic analysis. Enzyme analyses of fibroblasts, leukocytes, liver, or muscle are needed. The samples should be obtained as soon as possible after death to avoid postmortem changes [103]. However, autopsies are not always performed soon after death, so it is difficult to obtain fresh samples. In many forensic laboratories, frozen blood and organ samples preserved in phosphate-buffered formaldehyde solution are available, but frozen organ samples do not preserve well. A case was reported in which fibroblasts could be cultured on the fourth day postmortem [12]. This suggests that fibroblasts should be cultured as much possible in the future.

5. EXPANDED NEWBORN SCREENING

Some FAODs can be treated by avoiding fasting and glucose supplementation. However, effective therapy cannot be started until a definite diagnosis has been made. Delaying diagnosis by even a few days can lead to permanent mental retardation, coma, or sudden death. Early detection and early therapeutic intervention, especially during the asymptomatic period, are therefore important for patients and public health.

The Guthrie qualitative bacterial inhibition test was reported in the 1960s, which formed the basis for the first successful national neonatal screening programs for phenylketonuria (PKU) [104]. The testing for PKU in this way was the start of worldwide NBS.

NBS has been improved since the introduction of MS/MS. Millington et al. applied fast-atom bombardment MS/MS to NBS of IMDs in 1990 [105,106]. MS/MS eliminates the need for chromatographic separation, shortening analysis time to a few minutes. It can therefore handle a large number of samples simultaneously. Chace et al. validated this methodology for NBS of PKU and tyrosinemia by measuring phenylalanine and tyrosine in 1993 [107]. After that, validation for maple syrup urine disease (MSUD), homocystinuria, and MCAD deficiency were also reported [108-110]. Rashed et al. introduced electrospray ionization MS/MS to IMDs in 1994 [111,112], and a high throughput method for sample preparation and practical usage were developed in 1997 [113]. Since then, it has started to be used in NBS, as expanded NBS. Expanded NBS programs now cover a wide range of IMDs and are reported throughout the world: North America [114-117], Europe [118-120], Saudi Arabia [121], South Korea [122], Africa [123], and Australasia [124,125].

In Japan, the NBS Guthrie card is used for the detection of following diseases: PKU, MSUD, homocystinuria, galactosemia, congenital adrenal hyperplasia, and congenital hypothyroidism. Expanded NBS is only performed in restricted regions as a pilot study [52]. The NBS Guthrie cards for SUDI cases were retrospectively subjected to MS/MS analysis, which were consistent with FAODs [88]. If expanded NBS had been performed, they could have been diagnosed as FAODs, might have been successfully treated, and might have been able to prevent sudden death.

6. METABOLIC AUTOPSY IN PREGNANCY-RELATED CASES

Hypertension, elevated liver enzymes, and low platelets (HELLP) syndrome and acute fatty liver of pregnancy (AFLP) are said to be associated with LCHAD and MTP deficiencies [126]. Wilcken et al. reported this association in 1993, in which 11 pregnancies in five mothers (two of whom were already reported by Schoeman et al. in 1991 [127]) resulted in six babies with LCHAD deficiency [128]. The relationship between maternal liver diseases and other FAODs is controversial. A few reports describe the relationship between maternal liver diseases and some FAODs: CPT I [129,130], MCAD [131], and SCAD deficiencies [132].

The reason why FAOD in the fetus causes maternal disease remains to be fully clarified. Three sources (the heterozygous mother, the homozygous fetus, or the homozygous placenta) are candidates for potentially toxic intermediates. It is hypothesized that accumulated metabolic intermediates as free radicals may damage cell membranes and organelles. The damaged maternal endothelium may release inflammatory mediators and lead to multiple organ failure, in a similar manner to the pathophysiology of pre-eclampsia being damage to vascular endothelium [133,134].

Thus, not only SUDI cases but also pregnancy-related autopsy cases should be subjected to metabolic autopsy.

CONCLUSION

In this chapter we focus on the importance of metabolic autopsy and also emphasize the necessity of expanded NBS. We summarize fatty acid oxidation pathway and each disease of FAODs. FAODs are not common diseases among SUDI cases. However they are inherited in an autosomal recessive manner, and correct diagnosis and early detection are thus needed. Forensic scientists should routinely perform metabolic autopsy in SUDI cases and expanded NBS should be prevailingly available.

ACKNOWLEDGMENT

The authors thank Dr. P. Todd for revising English used in this article.

REFERENCES

[1] M. Hoffman. Scientific sleuths solve a murder mystery. *Science.* 254 (1991) 931.
[2] M.J. Bennett, P. Rinaldo. The metabolic autopsy comes of age. *Clin. Chem.* 47 (2001) 1145-1146.

[3] S.R. Limerick, C.J. Bacon. Terminology used by pathologists in reporting on sudden infant deaths. *J. Clin. Pathol.* 57 (2004) 309-311.

[4] S.J. Gould, M.A. Weber, N.J. Sebire. Variation and uncertainties in the classification of sudden unexpected infant deaths among paediatric pathologists in the UK: findings of a National Delphi Study. *J. Clin. Pathol.* 63 (2010) 796-799.

[5] R.L. Wilcox, C.C. Nelson, P. Stenzel, R.D. Steiner. Postmortem screening for fatty acid oxidation disorders by analysis of Guthrie cards with tandem mass spectrometry in sudden unexpected death in infancy. *J. Pediatr.* 141 (2002) 833-836.

[6] A. Cote, P. Russo, J. Michaud. Sudden unexpected deaths in infancy: what are the causes? *J. Pediatr.* 135 (1999) 437-443.

[7] C.M. Loughrey, M.A. Preece, A. Green. Sudden unexpected death in infancy (SUDI). *J. Clin. Pathol.* 58 (2005) 20-21.

[8] A. Cote. Investigating sudden unexpected death in infancy and early childhood. *Paediatr. Respir. Rev.* 11 (2010) 219-225.

[9] R.Y. Moon, R.S. Horne, F.R. Hauck. Sudden infant death syndrome. *Lancet.* 370 (2007) 1578-1587.

[10] M. Willinger, L.S. James, C. Catz. Defining the sudden infant death syndrome (SIDS): deliberations of an expert panel convened by the National Institute of Child Health and Human Development. *Pediatr. Pathol.* 11 (1991) 677-684.

[11] M.J. Bennett, S. Powell. Metabolic disease and sudden, unexpected death in infancy. *Hum. Pathol.* 25 (1994) 742-746.

[12] J.B. Lundemose, S. Kolvraa, N. Gregersen, E. Christensen, M. Gregersen. Fatty acid oxidation disorders as primary cause of sudden and unexpected death in infants and young children: an investigation performed on cultured fibroblasts from 79 children who died aged between 0-4 years. *Mol. Pathol.* 50 (1997) 212-217.

[13] R.G. Boles, E.A. Buck, M.G. Blitzer, M.S. Platt, T.M. Cowan, S.K. Martin, H. Yoon, J.A. Madsen, M. Reyes-Mugica, P. Rinaldo. Retrospective biochemical screening of fatty acid oxidation disorders in postmortem livers of 418 cases of sudden death in the first year of life. *J. Pediatr.* 132 (1998) 924-933.

[14] P. Rinaldo, H.R. Yoon, C. Yu, K. Raymond, C. Tiozzo, G. Giordano. Sudden and unexpected neonatal death: a protocol for the postmortem diagnosis of fatty acid oxidation disorders. *Semin. Perinatol.* 23 (1999) 204-210.

[15] D.H. Chace, J.C. DiPerna, B.L. Mitchell, B. Sgroi, L.F. Hofman, E.W. Naylor. Electrospray tandem mass spectrometry for analysis of acylcarnitines in dried postmortem blood specimens collected at autopsy from infants with unexplained cause of death. *Clin. Chem.* 47 (2001) 1166-1182.
[16] Y. Tamaoki, M. Kimura, Y. Hasegawa, M. Iga, M. Inoue, S. Yamaguchi. A survey of Japanese patients with mitochondrial fatty acid beta-oxidation and related disorders as detected from 1985 to 2000. *Brain. Dev.* 24 (2002) 675-680.
[17] P. Rinaldo, D. Matern, M.J. Bennett. Fatty acid oxidation disorders. *Annu. Rev. Physiol.* 64 (2002) 477-502.
[18] D. Moczulski, I. Majak, D. Mamczur. An overview of beta-oxidation disorders. *Postepy. Hig. Med. Dosw.* (Online.) 63 (2009) 266-277.
[19] K.G. Sim, J. Hammond, B. Wilcken. Strategies for the diagnosis of mitochondrial fatty acid beta-oxidation disorders. *Clin. Chim. Acta.* 323 (2002) 37-58.
[20] M. Kompare, W.B. Rizzo. Mitochondrial fatty-acid oxidation disorders. *Semin. Pediatr. Neurol.* 15 (2008) 140-149.
[21] W. Yu, X. Chu, G. Chen, D. Li. Studies of human mitochondrial 2,4-dienoyl-CoA reductase. *Arch. Biochem. Biophys.* 434 (2005) 195-200.
[22] S. DiMauro, P.M. DiMauro. Muscle carnitine palmityltransferase deficiency and myoglobinuria. *Science.* 182 (1973) 929-931.
[23] A. Koizumi, J. Nozaki, T. Ohura, T. Kayo, Y. Wada, J. Nezu, R. Ohashi, I. Tamai, Y. Shoji, G. Takada, S. Kibira, T. Matsuishi, A. Tsuji. Genetic epidemiology of the carnitine transporter OCTN2 gene in a Japanese population and phenotypic characterization in Japanese pedigrees with primary systemic carnitine deficiency. *Hum. Mol. Genet.* 8 (1999) 2247-2254.
[24] N. Longo, C. Amat di San Filippo, M. Pasquali. Disorders of carnitine transport and the carnitine cycle. *Am. J. Med. Genet. C. Semin. Med. Genet.* 142C (2006) 77-85.
[25] U. Spiekerkoetter, G. Huener, T. Baykal, M. Demirkol, M. Duran, R. Wanders, J. Nezu, E. Mayatepek. Silent and symptomatic primary carnitine deficiency within the same family due to identical mutations in the organic cation/carnitine transporter OCTN2. *J. Inherit. Metab. Dis.* 26 (2003) 613-615.
[26] J.P. Bonnefont, F. Djouadi, C. Prip-Buus, S. Gobin, A. Munnich, J. Bastin. Carnitine palmitoyltransferases 1 and 2: biochemical, molecular and medical aspects. *Mol. Aspects. Med.* 25 (2004) 495-520.

[27] P.F. Bougneres, J.M. Saudubray, C. Marsac, O. Bernard, M. Odievre, J. Girard. Fasting hypoglycemia resulting from hepatic carnitine palmitoyl transferase deficiency. *J. Pediatr.* 98 (1981) 742-746.

[28] G. Hug, S. Soukup, H. Berry, K. Bove. Carnitine palmityl transferase (CPT): deficiency of CPT II but not of CPT I with reduced total and free carnitine but increased acylcarnitine. *Pediat. Res.* 2 (1989) 115A.

[29] G. Hug, K.E. Bove, S. Soukup. Lethal neonatal multiorgan deficiency of carnitine palmitoyltransferase II. *N. Engl. J. Med.* 325 (1991) 1862-1864.

[30] A.B. Zinn, V.L. Zurcher, F. Kraus, C. Strohl, M.C. Walsh-Sukys, C.L. Hoppel. Carnitine palmitoyltransferase B (CPT B) deficiency: a heritable cause of neonatal cardiomyopathy and dysgenesis of the kidney. *Pediat. Res.* 29 (1991) 73A.

[31] F. Demaugre, J.P. Bonnefont, M. Colonna, C. Cepanec, J.P. Leroux, J.M. Saudubray. Infantile form of carnitine palmitoyltransferase II deficiency with hepatomuscular symptoms and sudden death. Physiopathological approach to carnitine palmitoyltransferase II deficiencies. *J. Clin. Invest.* 87 (1991) 859-864.

[32] J.P. Bonnefont, F. Demaugre, C. Prip-Buus, J.M. Saudubray, M. Brivet, N. Abadi, L. Thuillier. Carnitine palmitoyltransferase deficiencies. *Mol. Genet. Metab.* 68 (1999) 424-440.

[33] E. Sigauke, D. Rakheja, K. Kitson, M.J. Bennett. Carnitine palmitoyltransferase II deficiency: a clinical, biochemical, and molecular review. *Lab. Invest.* 83 (2003) 1543-1554.

[34] C.A. Stanley, D.E. Hale, G.T. Berry, S. Deleeuw, J. Boxer, J.P. Bonnefont. Brief report: a deficiency of carnitine-acylcarnitine translocase in the inner mitochondrial membrane. *N. Engl. J. Med.* 327 (1992) 19-23.

[35] M.E. Rubio-Gozalbo, J.A. Bakker, H.R. Waterham, R.J. Wanders. Carnitine-acylcarnitine translocase deficiency, clinical, biochemical and genetic aspects. *Mol. Aspects. Med.* 25 (2004) 521-532.

[36] T. Aoyama, Y. Uchida, R.I. Kelley, M. Marble, K. Hofman, J.H. Tonsgard, W.J. Rhead, T. Hashimoto. A novel disease with deficiency of mitochondrial very-long-chain acyl-CoA dehydrogenase. *Biochem. Biophys. Res. Commun.* 191 (1993) 1369-1372.

[37] C. Bertrand, C. Largilliere, M.T. Zabot, M. Mathieu, C. Vianey-Saban. Very long chain acyl-CoA dehydrogenase deficiency: identification of a new inborn error of mitochondrial fatty acid oxidation in fibroblasts. *Biochim. Biophys. Acta.* 1180 (1993) 327-329.

[38] S. Yamaguchi, Y. Indo, P.M. Coates, T. Hashimoto, K. Tanaka. Identification of very-long-chain acyl-CoA dehydrogenase deficiency in three patients previously diagnosed with long-chain acyl-CoA dehydrogenase deficiency. *Pediatr. Res.* 34 (1993) 111-113.

[39] B.S. Andresen, S. Olpin, B.J. Poorthuis, H.R. Scholte, C. Vianey-Saban, R. Wanders, L. IJlst, A. Morris, M. Pourfarzam, K. Bartlett, E.R. Baumgartner, J.B. deKlerk, L.D. Schroeder, T.J. Corydon, H. Lund, V. Winter, P. Bross, L. Bolund, N. Gregersen. Clear correlation of genotype with disease phenotype in very-long-chain acyl-CoA dehydrogenase deficiency. *Am. J. Hum. Genet.* 64 (1999) 479-494.

[40] T. Aoyama, M. Souri, S. Ushikubo, T. Kamijo, S. Yamaguchi, R.I. Kelley, W.J. Rhead, K. Uetake, K. Tanaka, T. Hashimoto. Purification of human very-long-chain acyl-coenzyme A dehydrogenase and characterization of its deficiency in seven patients. *J. Clin. Invest.* 95 (1995) 2465-2473.

[41] C. Largilliere, C. Vianey-Saban, M. Fontaine, C. Bertrand, N. Kacet, J.P. Farriaux. Mitochondrial very long chain acyl-CoA dehydrogenase deficiency -a new disorder of fatty acid oxidation. *Arch. Dis. Child. Fetal. Neonatal. Ed.* 73 (1995) F103-F105.

[42] K. Carpenter, R.J. Pollitt, B. Middleton. Human liver long-chain 3-hydroxyacyl-coenzyme A dehydrogenase is a multifunctional membrane-bound beta-oxidation enzyme of mitochondria. *Biochem. Biophys. Res. Commun.* 183 (1992) 443-448.

[43] Y. Uchida, K. Izai, T. Orii, T. Hashimoto. Novel fatty acid beta-oxidation enzymes in rat liver mitochondria. II. Purification and properties of enoyl-coenzyme A (CoA) hydratase/3-hydroxyacyl-CoA dehydrogenase/3-ketoacyl-CoA thiolase trifunctional protein. *J. Biol. Chem.* 267 (1992) 1034-1041.

[44] A.M. Das, S. Illsinger, T. Lucke, H. Hartmann, J.P. Ruiter, U. Steuerwald, H.R. Waterham, M. Duran, R.J. Wanders. Isolated mitochondrial long-chain ketoacyl-CoA thiolase deficiency resulting from mutations in the HADHB gene. *Clin. Chem.* 52 (2006) 530-534.

[45] R.J. Wanders, M. Duran, L. IJlst, J.P. de Jager, A.H. van Gennip, C. Jakobs, L. Dorland, F.J. van Sprang. Sudden infant death and long-chain 3-hydroxyacyl-CoA dehydrogenase. *Lancet.* 2 (1989) 52-53.

[46] R.J. Wanders, L. IJlst, A.H. van Gennip, C. Jakobs, J.P. de Jager, L. Dorland, F.J. van Sprang, M. Duran. Long-chain 3-hydroxyacyl-CoA dehydrogenase deficiency: identification of a new inborn error of

mitochondrial fatty acid beta-oxidation. *J. Inherit. Metab. Dis.* 13 (1990) 311-314.
[47] R.J. Wanders, L. IJlst, F. Poggi, J.P. Bonnefont, A. Munnich, M. Brivet, D. Rabier, J.M. Saudubray. Human trifunctional protein deficiency: a new disorder of mitochondrial fatty acid beta-oxidation. *Biochem. Biophys. Res. Commun.* 188 (1992) 1139-1145.
[48] S. Jackson, R.S. Kler, K. Bartlett, H. Briggs, L.A. Bindoff, M. Pourfarzam, D. Gardner-Medwin, D.M. Turnbull. Combined enzyme defect of mitochondrial fatty acid oxidation. *J. Clin. Invest.* 90 (1992) 1219-1225.
[49] T. Tyni, H. Pihko. Long-chain 3-hydroxyacyl-CoA dehydrogenase deficiency. *Acta. Paediatr.* 88 (1999) 237-245.
[50] M.E. den Boer, R.J. Wanders, A.A. Morris, L. IJlst, H.S. Heymans, F.A. Wijburg. Long-chain 3-hydroxyacyl-CoA dehydrogenase deficiency: clinical presentation and follow-up of 50 patients. *Pediatrics.* 109 (2002) 99-104.
[51] N. Gregersen, R. Lauritzen, K. Rasmussen. Suberylglycine excretion in the urine from a patient with dicarboxylic aciduria. *Clin. Chim. Acta.* 70 (1976) 417-425.
[52] Y. Shigematsu, S. Hirano, I. Hata, Y. Tanaka, M. Sudo, N. Sakura, T. Tajima, S. Yamaguchi. Newborn mass screening and selective screening using electrospray tandem mass spectrometry in Japan. *J. Chromatogr. B. Analyt. Technol. Biomed. Life. Sci.* 776 (2002) 39-48.
[53] S.D. Grosse, M.J. Khoury, C.L. Greene, K.S. Crider, R.J. Pollitt. The epidemiology of medium chain acyl-CoA dehydrogenase deficiency: an update. *Genet. Med.* 8 (2006) 205-212.
[54] A.J. Howat, M.J. Bennett, S. Variend, L. Shaw. Deficiency of medium chain fatty acylcoenzyme A dehydrogenase presenting as the sudden infant death syndrome. *Br. Med. J.* (Clin. Res. Ed.) 288 (1984) 976.
[55] A.J. Howat, M.J. Bennett, S. Variend, L. Shaw, P.C. Engel. Defects of metabolism of fatty acids in the sudden infant death syndrome. *Br. Med. J. (Clin. Res. Ed.)* 290 (1985) 1771-1773.
[56] T. Kamijo, Y. Indo, M. Souri, T. Aoyama, T. Hara, S. Yamamoto, S. Ushikubo, P. Rinaldo, I. Matsuda, A. Komiyama, T. Hashimoto. Medium chain 3-ketoacyl-coenzyme A thiolase deficiency: a new disorder of mitochondrial fatty acid beta-oxidation. *Pediatr. Res.* 42 (1997) 569-576.
[57] Tein, D.C. De Vivo, D.E. Hale, J.T. Clarke, H. Zinman, R. Laxer, A. Shore, S. DiMauro. Short-chain L-3-hydroxyacyl-CoA dehydrogenase

deficiency in muscle: a new cause for recurrent myoglobinuria and encephalopathy. *Ann. Neurol.* 30 (1991) 415-419.
[58] S.Y. Yang, X.Y. He, H. Schulz. 3-Hydroxyacyl-CoA dehydrogenase and short chain 3-hydroxyacyl-CoA dehydrogenase in human health and disease. *FEBS. J.* 272 (2005) 4874-4883.
[59] P.T. Clayton, S. Eaton, A. Aynsley-Green, M. Edginton, K. Hussain, S. Krywawych, V. Datta, H.E. Malingre, R. Berger, I.E. van den Berg. Hyperinsulinism in short-chain L-3-hydroxyacyl-CoA dehydrogenase deficiency reveals the importance of beta-oxidation in insulin secretion. *J. Clin. Invest.* 108 (2001) 457-465.
[60] D.M. Turnbull, K. Bartlett, D.L. Stevens, K.G. Alberti, G.J. Gibson, M.A. Johnson, A.J. McCulloch, H.S. Sherratt. Short-chain acyl-CoA dehydrogenase deficiency associated with a lipid-storage myopathy and secondary carnitine deficiency. *N. Engl. J. Med.* 311 (1984) 1232-1236.
[61] A. Bhala, S.M. Willi, P. Rinaldo, M.J. Bennett, E. Schmidt-Sommerfeld, D.E. Hale. Clinical and biochemical characterization of short-chain acyl-coenzyme A dehydrogenase deficiency. *J. Pediatr.* 126 (1995) 910-915.
[62] B.A. Amendt, C. Greene, L. Sweetman, J. Cloherty, V. Shih, A. Moon, L. Teel, W.J. Rhead. Short-chain acyl-coenzyme A dehydrogenase deficiency. Clinical and biochemical studies in two patients. *J. Clin. Invest.* 79 (1987) 1303-1309.
[63] B.T. van Maldegem, R.J. Wanders, F.A. Wijburg. Clinical aspects of short-chain acyl-CoA dehydrogenase deficiency. *J. Inherit. Metab. Dis.* 33 (2010) 507-511.
[64] R. Jethva, M.J. Bennett, J. Vockley. Short-chain acyl-coenzyme A dehydrogenase deficiency. *Mol. Genet. Metab.* 95 (2008) 195-200.
[65] J. Zhang, W. Zhang, D. Zou, G. Chen, T. Wan, M. Zhang, X. Cao. Cloning and functional characterization of ACAD-9, a novel member of human acyl-CoA dehydrogenase family. *Biochem. Biophys. Res. Commun.* 297 (2002) 1033-1042.
[66] M. He, S.L. Rutledge, D.R. Kelly, C.A. Palmer, G. Murdoch, N. Majumder, R.D. Nicholls, Z. Pei, P.A. Watkins, J. Vockley. A new genetic disorder in mitochondrial fatty acid beta-oxidation: ACAD9 deficiency. *Am. J. Hum. Genet.* 81 (2007) 87-103.
[67] R.K. Olsen, B.S. Andresen, E. Christensen, P. Bross, F. Skovby, N. Gregersen. Clear relationship between ETF/ETFDH genotype and phenotype in patients with multiple acyl-CoA dehydrogenation deficiency. *Hum. Mutat.* 22 (2003) 12-23.

[68] C.R. Roe, D.S. Millington, D.L. Norwood, N. Kodo, H. Sprecher, B.S. Mohammed, M. Nada, H. Schulz, R. McVie. 2,4-Dienoyl-coenzyme A reductase deficiency: a possible new disorder of fatty acid oxidation. *J. Clin. Invest.* 85 (1990) 1703-1707.

[69] J. Vockley, D.A. Whiteman. Defects of mitochondrial beta-oxidation: a growing group of disorders. *Neuromuscul. Disord.* 12 (2002) 235-246.

[70] R.D. Reye, G. Morgan, J. Baral. Encephalopathy and fatty degeneration of the viscera. A disease entity in childhood. *Lancet.* 2 (1963) 749-752.

[71] A. Pugliese, T. Beltramo, D. Torre. Reye's and Reye's-like syndromes. *Cell. Biochem. Funct.* 26 (2008) 741-746.

[72] B. Sinclair-Smith, F. Dinsdale, J. Emery. Evidence of duration and type of illness in children found unexpectedly dead. *Arch. Dis. Child.* 51 (1976) 424-429.

[73] T. Sawaguchi, H. Nishida. Fatty liver in sudden infant death autopsies. *Am. J. Forensic. Med. Pathol.* 19 (1998) 294.

[74] Z. Yang, P.E. Lantz, J.A. Ibdah. Post-mortem analysis for two prevalent beta-oidation mutations in sudden infant death. *Pediatr. Int.* 49 (2007) 883-887.

[75] L.L. Bieber, Y.R. Choi. Isolation and identification of aliphatic short-chain acylcarnitines from beef heart: possible role for carnitine in branched-chain amino acid metabolism. *Proc. Natl. Acad. Sci. U. S. A.* 74 (1977) 2795-2798.

[76] C.R. Roe, C.L. Hoppel, T.E. Stacey, R.A. Chalmers, B.M. Tracey, D.S. Millington. Metabolic response to carnitine in methylmalonic aciduria. An effective strategy for elimination of propionyl groups. *Arch. Dis. Child.* 58 (1983) 916-920.

[77] D.H. Chace. Mass spectrometry in the clinical laboratory. *Chem. Rev.* 101 (2001) 445-477.

[78] M.J. Bennett, M.C. Ragni, I. Hood, D.E. Hale. Comparison of postmortem urinary and vitreous-humor organic-acids. *Ann. Clin. Biochem.* 29 (1992) 541-545.

[79] R.G. Boles, S.K. Martin, M.G. Blitzer, P. Rinaldo. Biochemical diagnosis of fatty acid oxidation disorders by metabolite analysis of postmortem liver. *Hum. Pathol.* 25 (1994) 735-741.

[80] M.S. Rashed, P.T. Ozand, M.J. Bennett, J.J. Barnard, D.R. Govindaraju, P. Rinaldo. Inborn errors of metabolism diagnosed in sudden death cases by acylcarnitine analysis of postmortem bile. *Clin. Chem.* 41 (1995) 1109-1114.

[81] P.M. Kemp, B.B. Little, R.O. Bost, D.B. Dawson. Whole blood levels of dodecanoic acid, a routinely detectable forensic marker for a genetic disease often misdiagnosed as sudden infant death syndrome (SIDS): MCAD deficiency. *Am. J. Forensic. Med. Pathol.* 17 (1996) 79-82.

[82] P. Rinaldo, C.A. Stanley, B.Y. Hsu, L.A. Sanchez, H.J. Stern. Sudden neonatal death in carnitine transporter deficiency. *J. Pediatr.* 131 (1997) 304-305.

[83] J.B. Holton, J.T. Allen, C.A. Green, S. Partington, R.E. Gilbert, P.J. Berry. Inherited metabolic diseases in the sudden infant death syndrome. *Arch. Dis. Child.* 66 (1991) 1315-1317.

[84] M.E. Miller, J.G. Brooks, N. Forbes, R. Insel. Frequency of medium-chain acyl-CoA dehydrogenase deficiency G-985 mutation in sudden infant death syndrome. *Pediatr. Res. 31* (1992) 305-307.

[85] R. Arens, D. Gozal, K. Jain, S. Muscati, E.T. Heuser, J.C. Williams, T.G. Keens, S.L. Ward. Prevalence of medium-chain acyl-coenzyme A dehydrogenase deficiency in the sudden infant death syndrome. *J. Pediatr.* 122 (1993) 715-718.

[86] B. Lemieux, R. Giguere, D. Cyr, D. Shapcott, M. McCann, M. Tuchman. Screening urine of 3-week-old newborns: lack of association between sudden infant death syndrome and some metabolic disorders. *Pediatrics.* 91 (1993) 986-988.

[87] R. Fingerhut, W. Roschinger, A.C. Muntau, T. Dame, J. Kreischer, R. Arnecke, A. Superti-Furga, H. Troxler, B. Liebl, B. Olgemoller, A.A. Roscher. Hepatic carnitine palmitoyltransferase I deficiency: acylcarnitine profiles in blood spots are highly specific. *Clin. Chem.* 47 (2001) 1763-1768.

[88] T. Yamamoto, H. Tanaka, H. Kobayashi, K. Okamura, T. Tanaka, Y. Emoto, K. Sugimoto, M. Nakatome, N. Sakai, H. Kuroki, S. Yamaguchi, R. Matoba. Retrospective review of Japanese sudden unexpected death in infancy: The importance of metabolic autopsy and expanded newborn screening. *Mol. Genet. Metab.* 102 (2011) 399-406.

[89] S.E. Olpin. The metabolic investigation of sudden infant death. *Ann. Clin. Biochem.* 41 (2004) 282-293.

[90] F. Taroni, E. Verderio, S. Fiorucci, P. Cavadini, G. Finocchiaro, G. Uziel, E. Lamantea, C. Gellera, S. DiDonato. Molecular characterization of inherited carnitine palmitoyltransferase II deficiency. *Proc. Natl. Acad. Sci. U. S. A.* 89 (1992) 8429-8433.

[91] K. Wataya, J. Akanuma, P. Cavadini, Y. Aoki, S. Kure, F. Invernizzi, I. Yoshida, J. Kira, F. Taroni, Y. Matsubara, K. Narisawa. Two CPT2

mutations in three Japanese patients with carnitine palmitoyltransferase II deficiency: functional analysis and association with polymorphic haplotypes and two clinical phenotypes. *Hum. Mutat.* 11 (1998) 377-386.

[92] Y. Chen, H. Mizuguchi, D. Yao, M. Ide, Y. Kuroda, Y. Shigematsu, S. Yamaguchi, M. Yamaguchi, M. Kinoshita, H. Kido. Thermolabile phenotype of carnitine palmitoyltransferase II variations as a predisposing factor for influenza-associated encephalopathy. *FEBS. Lett.* 579 (2005) 2040-2044.

[93] D. Yao, H. Mizuguchi, M. Yamaguchi, H. Yamada, J. Chida, K. Shikata, H. Kido. Thermal instability of compound variants of carnitine palmitoyltransferase II and impaired mitochondrial fuel utilization in influenza-associated encephalopathy. *Hum. Mutat.* 29 (2008) 718-727.

[94] R.J. Smeets, J.A. Smeitink, B.A. Semmekrot, H.R. Scholte, R.J. Wanders, L.P. van den Heuvel. A novel splice site mutation in neonatal carnitine palmitoyltransferase II deficiency. *J. Hum. Genet.* 48 (2003) 8-13.

[95] M. Deschauer, Z.M. Chrzanowska-Lightowlers, E. Biekmann, M. Pourfarzam, R.W. Taylor, D.M. Turnbull, S. Zierz. A splice junction mutation in muscle carnitine palmitoyltransferase II deficiency. *Mol. Genet. Metab.* 79 (2003) 124-128.

[96] N. Gregersen, B.S. Andresen, M.J. Corydon, T.J. Corydon, R.K. Olsen, L. Bolund, P. Bross. Mutation analysis in mitochondrial fatty acid oxidation defects: Exemplified by acyl-CoA dehydrogenase deficiencies, with special focus on genotype-phenotype relationship. *Hum. Mutat.* 18 (2001) 169-189.

[97] Y. Ohashi, Y. Hasegawa, K. Murayama, M. Ogawa, T. Hasegawa, M. Kawai, N. Sakata, K. Yoshida, H. Yarita, K. Imai, I. Kumagai, K. Murakami, H. Hasegawa, S. Noguchi, I. Nonaka, S. Yamaguchi, I. Nishino. A new diagnostic test for VLCAD deficiency using immunohistochemistry. *Neurology.* 62 (2004) 2209-2213.

[98] S. Ushikubo, T. Aoyama, T. Kamijo, R.J. Wanders, P. Rinaldo, J. Vockley, T. Hashimoto. Molecular characterization of mitochondrial trifunctional protein deficiency: formation of the enzyme complex is important for stabilization of both alpha- and beta-subunits. *Am. J. Hum. Genet.* 58 (1996) 979-988.

[99] K.E. Orii, T. Aoyama, K. Wakui, Y. Fukushima, H. Miyajima, S. Yamaguchi, T. Orii, N. Kondo, T. Hashimoto. Genomic and mutational analysis of the mitochondrial trifunctional protein beta-subunit

(HADHB) gene in patients with trifunctional protein deficiency. *Hum. Mol. Genet.* 6 (1997) 1215-1224.

[100] L. IJlst, R.J. Wanders, S. Ushikubo, T. Kamijo, T. Hashimoto. Molecular basis of long-chain 3-hydroxyacyl-CoA dehydrogenase deficiency: identification of the major disease-causing mutation in the alpha-subunit of the mitochondrial trifunctional protein. *Biochim. Biophys. Acta.* 1215 (1994) 347-350.

[101] J. Purevsuren, T. Fukao, Y. Hasegawa, S. Fukuda, H. Kobayashi, S. Yamaguchi. Study of deep intronic sequence exonization in a Japanese neonate with a mitochondrial trifunctional protein deficiency. *Mol. Genet. Metab.* 95 (2008) 46-51.

[102] N. Gregersen, V.S. Winter, M.J. Corydon, T.J. Corydon, P. Rinaldo, A. Ribes, G. Martinez, M.J. Bennett, C. Vianey-Saban, A. Bhala, D.E. Hale, W. Lehnert, S. Kmoch, M. Roig, E. Riudor, H. Eiberg, B.S. Andresen, P. Bross, L.A. Bolund, S. Kolvraa. Identification of four new mutations in the short-chain acyl-CoA dehydrogenase (SCAD) gene in two patients: one of the variant alleles, 511C->T, is present at an unexpectedly high frequency in the general population, as was the case for 625G->A, together conferring susceptibility to ethylmalonic aciduria. *Hum. Mol. Genet.* 7 (1998) 619-627.

[103] L.M. Ernst, N. Sondheimer, M.A. Deardorff, M.J. Bennett, B.R. Pawel. The value of the metabolic autopsy in the pediatric hospital setting. *J. Pediatr.* 148 (2006) 779-783.

[104] R. Guthrie, A. Susi. A simple phenylalanine method for detecting phenylketonuria in large populations of newborn infants. *Pediatrics.* 32 (1963) 338-343.

[105] D.S. Millington, N. Kodo, D.L. Norwood, C.R. Roe. Tandem mass spectrometry: a new method for acylcarnitine profiling with potential for neonatal screening for inborn errors of metabolism. *J. Inherit. Metab. Dis.* 13 (1990) 321-324.

[106] D.S. Millington, N. Kodo, N. Terada, D. Roe, D.H. Chace. The analysis of diagnostic markers of genetic disorders in human blood and urine using tandem mass spectrometry with liquid secondary ion mass spectrometry. *Int. J. Mass. Spectrom.* 111 (1991) 211-228.

[107] D.H. Chace, D.S. Millington, N. Terada, S.G. Kahler, C.R. Roe, L.F. Hofman. Rapid diagnosis of phenylketonuria by quantitative analysis for phenylalanine and tyrosine in neonatal blood spots by tandem mass spectrometry. *Clin. Chem.* 39 (1993) 66-71.

[108] D.H. Chace, S.L. Hillman, D.S. Millington, S.G. Kahler, C.R. Roe, E.W. Naylor. Rapid diagnosis of maple syrup urine disease in blood spots from newborns by tandem mass spectrometry. *Clin. Chem.* 41 (1995) 62-68.

[109] D.H. Chace, S.L. Hillman, D.S. Millington, S.G. Kahler, B.W. Adam, H.L. Levy. Rapid diagnosis of homocystinuria and other hypermethioninemias from newborns' blood spots by tandem mass spectrometry. *Clin. Chem.* 42 (1996) 349-355.

[110] D.H. Chace, S.L. Hillman, J.L. Van Hove, E.W. Naylor. Rapid diagnosis of MCAD deficiency: quantitative analysis of octanoylcarnitine and other acylcarnitines in newborn blood spots by tandem mass spectrometry. *Clin. Chem.* 43 (1997) 2106-2113.

[111] M.S. Rashed, P.T. Ozand, M.E. Harrison, P.J.F. Watkins, S. Evans. Electrospray tandem mass-spectrometry in the diagnosis of organic acidemias. *Rapid. Commun. Mass. Spectrom.* 8 (1994) 129-133.

[112] M.S. Rashed, P.T. Ozand, M.P. Bucknall, D. Little. Diagnosis of inborn errors of metabolism from blood spots by acylcarnitines and amino acids profiling using automated electrospray tandem mass spectrometry. *Pediatr. Res.* 38 (1995) 324-331.

[113] M.S. Rashed, M.P. Bucknall, D. Little, A. Awad, M. Jacob, M. Alamoudi, M. Alwattar, P.T. Ozand. Screening blood spots for inborn errors of metabolism by electrospray tandem mass spectrometry with a microplate batch process and a computer algorithm for automated flagging of abnormal profiles. *Clin. Chem.* 43 (1997) 1129-1141.

[114] T.H. Zytkovicz, E.F. Fitzgerald, D. Marsden, C.A. Larson, V.E. Shih, D.M. Johnson, A.W. Strauss, A.M. Comeau, R.B. Eaton, G.F. Grady. Tandem mass spectrometric analysis for amino, organic, and fatty acid disorders in newborn dried blood spots: a two-year summary from the New England Newborn Screening Program. *Clin. Chem.* 47 (2001) 1945-1955.

[115] S. Albers, S.E. Waisbren, M.G. Ampola, T.G. Brewster, L.W. Burke, L.A. Demmer, J. Filiano, R.M. Greenstein, C.L. Ingham, M.S. Korson, D. Marsden, R.C. Schwartz, M.R. Seashore, V.E. Shih, H.L. Levy. New England Consortium: a model for medical evaluation of expanded newborn screening with tandem mass spectrometry. *J. Inherit. Metab. Dis.* 24 (2001) 303-304.

[116] D.M. Frazier, D.S. Millington, S.E. McCandless, D.D. Koeberl, S.D. Weavil, S.H. Chaing, J. Muenzer. The tandem mass spectrometry

newborn screening experience in North Carolina: 1997-2005. *J. Inherit. Metab. Dis.* 29 (2006) 76-85.
[117] B.L. Therrell, J. Adams. Newborn screening in North America. *J. Inherit. Metab. Dis.* 30 (2007) 447-465.
[118] A. Schulze, M. Lindner, D. Kohlmuller, K. Olgemoller, E. Mayatepek, G.F. Hoffmann. Expanded newborn screening for inborn errors of metabolism by electrospray ionization-tandem mass spectrometry: results, outcome, and implications. *Pediatrics.* 111 (2003) 1399-1406.
[119] J.G. Loeber. Neonatal screening in Europe; the situation in 2004. *J. Inherit. Metab. Dis.* 30 (2007) 430-438.
[120] O.A. Bodamer, G.F. Hoffmann, M. Lindner. Expanded newborn screening in Europe 2007. *J. Inherit. Metab. Dis.* 30 (2007) 439-444.
[121] M.S. Rashed. Clinical applications of tandem mass spectrometry: ten years of diagnosis and screening for inherited metabolic diseases. J. Chromatogr. *B. Biomed. Sci. Appl.* 758 (2001) 27-48.
[122] H.R. Yoon, K.R. Lee, S. Kang, D.H. Lee, H.W. Yoo, W.K. Min, D.H. Cho, S.M. Shin, J. Kim, J. Song, H.J. Yoon, S. Seo, S.H. Hahn. Screening of newborns and high-risk group of children for inborn metabolic disorders using tandem mass spectrometry in South Korea: a three-year report. *Clin. Chim. Acta.* 354 (2005) 167-180.
[123] A.A. Saadallah, M.S. Rashed. Newborn screening: experiences in the Middle East and North Africa. *J. Inherit. Metab. Dis.* 30 (2007) 482-489.
[124] V. Wiley, K. Carpenter, B. Wilcken. Newborn screening with tandem mass spectrometry: 12 months' experience in NSW Australia. *Acta. Paediatr. Suppl.* 88 (1999) 48-51.
[125] B. Wilcken, V. Wiley, J. Hammond, K. Carpenter. Screening newborns for inborn errors of metabolism by tandem mass spectrometry. *N. Engl. J. Med.* 348 (2003) 2304-2312.
[126] P.S. Shekhawat, D. Matern, A.W. Strauss. Fetal fatty acid oxidation disorders, their effect on maternal health and neonatal outcome: impact of expanded newborn screening on their diagnosis and management. *Pediatr. Res.* 57 (2005) 78R-86R.
[127] M.N. Schoeman, R.G. Batey, B. Wilcken. Recurrent acute fatty liver of pregnancy associated with a fatty-acid oxidation defect in the offspring. *Gastroenterology.* 100 (1991) 544-548.
[128] B. Wilcken, K.C. Leung, J. Hammond, R. Kamath, J.V. Leonard. Pregnancy and fetal long-chain 3-hydroxyacyl coenzyme A dehydrogenase deficiency. *Lancet.* 341 (1993) 407-408.

[129] A.M. Innes, L.E. Seargeant, K. Balachandra, C.R. Roe, R.J. Wanders, J.P. Ruiter, O. Casiro, D.A. Grewar, C.R. Greenberg. Hepatic carnitine palmitoyltransferase I deficiency presenting as maternal illness in pregnancy. *Pediatr. Res.* 47 (2000) 43-45.

[130] K. Ylitalo, T. Vanttinen, E. Halmesmaki, T. Tyni. Serious pregnancy complications in a patient with previously undiagnosed carnitine palmitoyltransferase 1 deficiency. *Am. J. Obstet. Gynecol.* 192 (2005) 2060-2062.

[131] J. Nelson, B. Lewis, B. Walters. The HELLP syndrome associated with fetal medium-chain acyl-CoA dehydrogenase deficiency. *J. Inherit. Metab. Dis.* 23 (2000) 518-519.

[132] D. Matern, P. Hart, A.P. Murtha, J. Vockley, N. Gregersen, D.S. Millington, W.R. Treem. Acute fatty liver of pregnancy associated with short-chain acyl-coenzyme A dehydrogenase deficiency. *J. Pediatr.* 138 (2001) 585-588.

[133] D. Rakheja, M.J. Bennett, B.B. Rogers. Long-chain L-3-hydroxyacyl-coenzyme a dehydrogenase deficiency: a molecular and biochemical review. *Lab. Invest.* 82 (2002) 815-824.

[134] J.A. Ibdah. Acute fatty liver of pregnancy: an update on pathogenesis and clinical implications. *World. J. Gastroenterol.* 12 (2006) 7397-7404.

Chapter 2

CHALLENGING THE AUTHORITY OF THE AUTOPSY IN CORONIAL INVESTIGATIONS

Belinda Carpenter, Gordon Tait, Michael Barnes and Charles Naylor
School of Justice Studies, Faculty of Law, QUT,
Queensland, Australia

ABSTRACT

The central purpose of this chapter is to address the tension between legal and medical discourses within the coronial/medico-legal system. In the context of a death investigation, medical expertise, manifest through the knowledge gained in an internal autopsy, is positioned as contributing the more valuable facts of the case, especially when contrasted with the evidence gathered at the scene of the death. We challenge this taken for granted understanding of medical knowledge in three ways: first, we examine the aspects of the history, philosophy and consequences of the processes by which the medical model gained its current dominance; second, we challenge the assumption that internal autopsy adds value to the death investigation, by utilising data from our own research in Australia; and finally, we engage with the debate about the purpose of a coronial/medico-legal investigation and role of an internal autopsy within that system.

1. INTRODUCTION: THE CORONIAL INVESTIGATION AS A CONTESTED SITE

The role of the coroner is to preside over death investigations for where there is a suspicion as to cause of death, a need to identify the identity of the deceased, a death of unknown cause or a violent or unnatural death.[1] In more recent times coroners have also been required to preside over deaths which occur in institutions, including prisons and aged care facilities. They are aided in their investigatory work by police, who visit the scene of the death and gather relevant information from the scene, and pathologists and other medical personnel who perform autopsies and other medical procedures on the deceased. They are responsible for a cause of death certificate being determined and recorded in the Registry of Births Deaths and Marriages.

All coronial systems require some form of autopsy once the deceased has been ascertained as a reportable death. Autopsies in the coronial system take three forms: external viewing of the body, a partial internal autopsy, and a full internal autopsy. In the Coronial systems of Australia, New Zealand, England and Wales, internal autopsies predominate.[2] This focus on internal autopsies as the key tool in any coronial investigation of death indicates that, in these coronial systems at least, there is an assumption that internal autopsies will always add value to a death investigation. This chapter will address how this assumption came about, and whether it can be regarded as valid.

However, examination of this issue requires consideration of a broader, quite seminal question about the purpose of an autopsy within a coronial death investigation. Terms such as "cause of death" or "how the person died" are imprecise and to some extent open ended. Moreover, coroners, who are predominantly legally trained, and pathologists, who are medical professionals, embrace different epistemologies, use different methods and have not communicated sufficiently to have developed a shared consensus about exactly what coronial investigations are meant to achieve. In these circumstances it should not be surprising they have different views about the value of internal autopsies in coronial investigations. We follow Freckleton in suggesting that the relationship between coroners and institutes of forensic

---

[1] Bierig, J. "Informed Consent in the Practice of Pathology." Archives of Pathology and Laboratory Medicine, 125, no.11 (2001): 1425-1429.
[2] Luce T, Death Certification and Investigation in England, Wales and Northern Ireland: The Report of a Fundamental Review (Crown Copyright, 2003) p 19; Smith J, The Shipman Inquiry. Third Report – Death Certification and the Investigation of Deaths by Coroners (Command Paper CM 5854, 2003) p v.

medicine "has the potential to be extremely constructive [but] also has the potential for tension."[3]

2. WHY DOES MEDICINE DOMINATE THE CORONIAL PROCESS?

There are a wide variety of reasons for the apparent supremacy of medical over legal discourses with the Coronial system, however this chapter will only focus on two. The first involves a brief historical explanation of the forces that shaped the role of Coroner, while the second examines a philosophical issue regarding the intellectual hegemony held by science and medicine within the logic of modernity.

a.) History and the Coroner

It is generally agreed that the modern coronial system has its origins in England in 1194 'when the Justices in Eyre were required to see that three knights and one clerk were elected in every county as "keepers of the pleas of the crown"'.[4] Despite the implications of his formal title, the 'crown pleas' for which the Coroner became responsible, focused primarily upon those related to sudden or unexpected deaths and the felonies of homicide and suicide. Significantly, the appointment of the Coroner at this time, it is argued, was in the interests of good order, justice and, most importantly, royal revenue. Certainly, Richard I was in desperate need of money, and as Knapman notes, the judicial functions of the Coroner were of secondary importance to revenue gathering—a task for which the existing office of Sheriff was regarded as unsuitable.[5]

By the middle of the 13th century, the identity of the county Coroner was well established, and the Coroner was the only person who could carry out an investigation on a dead body. The body had to be viewed prior to an inquest being held, and an inquest could not be held unless there was a body. Even with this crucial role, the position of the Coroner eventually began to decline

---

[3] Ian Freckleton (2007) "Death Investigation, the coroner and therapeutic jurisprudence" Journal of Law and Medicine, 15, p249
[4] Hunnisett, R. The Medieval Coroner. WMW. Gaunt & Sons, Inc.: Florida (1961): 1.
[5] Knapman, P. "The crowner's quest." Journal of the Royal Society of Medicine. 86, (1993): 716.

in importance due to the rise of a parallel legal office—the Justice of the Peace—such that by 1500 the sole remaining function performed by the Coroner was the holding of inquests into violent deaths.[6] Tension continued to exist between these two positions for the next three hundred years, and it was only resolved with the Births and Deaths Registration Act 1836 (UK), which formalised the legal obligations of Coroners, and provided for the registration of every death taking place in England and Wales. According to Freckleton and Ranson, this legislation also 'recognised that the jurisdiction of the Coroner was far wider than just the investigation of violent deaths',[7] since it required the collection and recording of accurate statistical information about mortality, placing specific duties on Coroners to report all deaths.[8]

By the end of the 19th century, the role of the Coroner was becoming more like the modern Coroner of the 21st century as the result of further legislative changes. For example, the establishment of the Coroners Act 1887 (UK) removed the last link between the Coroner and the financial interests of the sovereign, conceptualising the role instead as 'providing a means of investigating the circumstances and causes of deaths, where it was in the public interest that there be an investigation', which remains the statutory basis of the law today.[9]

Importantly, for the purposes of this discussion, the Coroners (Amendment) Act 1926 (UK) increased the power of Coroners to order autopsies for both natural and unnatural deaths without the need for an inquest. This legislation defined their qualifications as having to be either medical or legal, as well as positioning the role of Coroner more as information gathering than criminal detection. Indeed, by the end of the nineteenth century, the investigative work conducted by the Coroner to provide evidence for inquests was delegated to the police force who undertook these tasks under the direction of the Coroner. Finally, coronial juries were no longer to be mandatory. Not only did this discontinue the practice of the Coroner summonsing juries for inquests, but it also established a lesser reliance on the lay perspectives of the public that constituted these juries.[10]

---

[6] ibid., 719.
[7] Freckelton, I. and Ranson, D. Death investigation and the Coroner's inquest. Victoria: Oxford University Press, (2006):15.
[8] Plueckhahn, V. D. Ethics, legal medicine and forensic pathology. Melbourne: Melbourne University Press, (1983):98.
[9] Freckleton, I. and Ranson, D. (2006):21.
[10] ibid, 49-50.

It has been argued that these changes signalled the start of a long struggle over the role of Coroner.[11] That is, medicine began a struggle for dominance against a much older forms of organisation and sets of truth-claims—largely those of the wider citizenry, manifest in the forms of the elected jury, and the legal review of evidence within the public hearing. Burney cited the fascinating example of the contest in 1830 between two candidates for the office of county Coroner, one a surgeon and the other a lawyer. The surgeon, Thomas Wakely, under the banner 'Reason and Science against Ignorance and Prejudice', sought to introduce 'enlightenment' to proceedings normally 'fettered by legal sophistry and precedents'.[12] In opposition, the supporters of the lawyer William Baker, characterised medical knowledge, not as adding a new form of objective truth to the proceedings, but as an exclusory, undemocratic form of intervention that imposed itself on the inquest, immune from the challenge of anyone but other doctors. If the Coroner were to be a doctor, it was argued, they would, 'draw the attention of the jury from the plain and straightforward investigation of the facts, into the labyrinths of his own scientific investigations'.[13]

The contrast between these respective campaigns highlights the differences that still exist between the two different knowledge-bases, and their underlying claims for professional supremacy within the context of the coronial investigation. Arguably the complex information produced by the contemporary autopsy—the 'labyrinths' of scientific investigation—constitute precisely the kind of exclusory truth-claim referred to above, truth-claims which have come to supersede the processes and practices of information gathering and assessment from the scene of the death, as characterised by the traditional review of evidence (and latterly, police evidence) at a public hearing.

The development of the office of the coroner has been dealt with in some detail here because its history shapes the way the role is discharged today. Coroners developed as, and remain, an organ of civil society designed to scrutinise sudden, unnatural, violent or wrongful deaths, especially in state custody, using open, transparent and participatory methods that give due weight to the interests and opinions of those most affected by the death. The positioning of the coroner as part of the third and most independent arm of government means it is inevitably political: coroners' findings impact

---

[11] Burney, I. Bodies of Evidence: medicine and the politics of the English Inquest, 1830-1926. John Hopkins University: Baltimore (2000).
[12] ibid, 18.
[13] ibid, 19.

government policy and the allocation of public resources. An adherence to an epistemology that blends inquisitorial and therapeutic jurisprudence with a more traditional adjudicative function distinguishes coronial proceedings from both the rest of the legal system and from forensic pathology.

The questions now arises: why is that the information produced by the scientific autopsy is given such a pre-eminent status in the truth-gathering process, in comparison to the more prosaic practices of death-scene investigation, and is this pre-eminence warranted? The answers to these questions are more philosophical in nature, and lie in the logic of modernity.

b.) Science, Truth and Modernity

In Burney's analysis, he notes the importance of the notion of expertise within the debates over the control of the coronial investigation, and also more generally as a fundamental component of modern governance.[14] He is not alone in making these observations, as a wide range of other writers have pointed to the significance of expertise within modern government, particularly those writing on the rise of liberalism. Burchell argues that liberalism took as its central problem the demarcation of those areas of necessary state intervention from those of autonomy.[15] However, large portions of society were not just to be left to their own devices, instead liberalism adopted far less direct forms of management, such as the recruitment of experts to act as relays between the piecemeal agencies of government and various target populations. In doing so, the modernist state did not seek to manage conduct based solely upon such clumsy coercive mechanisms as laws, decrees and regulations, rather it administered the citizenry through the expertise associated with disciplines like medicine, family guidance, welfare, psychology, counselling and pedagogy.[16]

Modernity is generally regarded as arriving around the time of the Enlightenment in the 17th century, and is most frequently characterised as an era dominated by the underpinning belief that, through the use of reason, it would be possible to solve all the problems of humanity. With its mantra of

---

[14] ibid, 11.
[15] Burchell, G. "Liberal Government and Techniques of the Self". Economy and Society. 22, no.3 (1993): 267–283.
[16] Gordon, C. "Governmental Rationality: An Introduction." In The Foucault Effect: Studies in Governmentality, eds. G. Burchell, C. Gordon and P. Miller, London: Harvester Wheatsheaf, (1991); Rose, N. "Government, Authority and Expertise in Advanced Liberalism," Economy and Society. 22, no.3 (1993): 283–299.

truth, objectivity and progress, modernity had arrived, the dark ages had ended, and humanity had come of age. This optimistic vision of modernity was a set of narratives taken up in many different sectors of society, with probably the greatest advocate, and exemplar, of modernist thinking being science. With the exception of a few notable heretics,[17] science has long been its own best publicist, cordoning off the rights to the production of truth, and anointing itself as the vanguard of society's inexorable journey into a better future.

This notion of objectivity forms one of the central pillars within the logic of modernity, and the new forms of expertise that developed within it have succeeded, in large part, because of the status of the truth claims they produce:

> 'Experts' are key figures in the history and historiography of the modern state, in large part because the convergence between their model of knowledge making and the increasing stress placed on disinterestedness as the legitimating grounds for governmental action. Expert authority operates on the basis of detachment ...[18]

It would seem apparent that the current reliance on full internal autopsies most likely rests on this very detachment, a perceived necessary objectivity that legal investigation is deemed to lack. Medical investigation rests only on the facts of the death, gained through a thorough investigation of the internal organs of the deceased. In such situations, the medical investigation appears less open to interpretation and more scientifically supportable, that is, it is grounded in a belief in the objective fact finding nature of scientific investigation. In contrast, legal investigation is seen to largely rely upon the subjective opinions of family and friends, as well as the circumstantial evidence gathered at the scene, which may include a suicide note, empty packets of medication, or knowledge that the house was secure. Within the logic of modernity, these are widely regarded as inferior mechanisms of truth-assessment.

The pertinent issue here is that the notion of 'objectivity', and the status of the truth claims produced by its scientific exemplars, may be significantly more problematic than popular ideology suggests. For example, Feyerabend suggests that a number of qualifications should be placed upon the claims made by science, two of which are worthy of mention here.[19] First, he argues that the relatively uncritical acceptance of scientific truths is based upon a

---

[17] Popper, K. The Logic of Scientific Discovery, (London: Hutchinson, 1959); Feyerabend, P. Against Method. London: Verso, (1975).
[18] Burney, (2000), 8.
[19] Feyerabend, P. Science in a Free society. Verso: London, (1978).

belief in its infallibility, and the notion that it can prove its claims. Science is simply regarded as the most efficient means available for 'uncovering' truth, based in the fair, rigorous and controlled scientific method. However, Feyerabend argues that the 'rigorous' scientific method is, in practical terms, generally nebulous collection of rules and procedures, often applied unevenly and pragmatically.

Second, and part of the reason the scientific method is no magical guarantor of truth, is that science is a social process, and the truths it produces are forged within specific social contexts, and Feyerabend is far from alone in making this assertion. Collins also challenges the common assumption that scientific endeavours are somehow independent from human intentionality, contending instead that social factors exert a considerable influence upon the nature, course and success of scientific practice.[20] Collins stresses the importance of networks of communication between scientists, the tacit knowledge necessary to succeed in certain areas, and the mechanics by which one theory, or set of practices, gains ascendency over another.

Several points are worthy of note here: first, the scientific autopsy does not immediately translate into the necessary production of medical truth, and from there to a concomitant clear and infallible answer to all the questions raised in the coronial investigation. Like the investigation at the scene of death, the autopsy itself is a social process, where specific pieces of information are selected over other, choices are made, ideas exchanged and conclusions drawn. Truth does not emerge, full formed and mature, with pathologists as mere spectators. Second, much of the information produced through the autopsy, whether true or otherwise, adds little to the coronial process. It is a testament to the modernist belief in scientific truth-making that if answers are to be found anywhere, then they are more likely to be produced by the status-laden expertise of medicine, rather than the significantly less valorised forms of expertise associated with law enforcement agencies. Finally, there is the assumption that even if other forms of non-scientific truth are useful in their own way, they require the ultimate seal of certainty provided by the autopsy. Indeed, why not let the pathologist have access to the body— the argument runs—when it will allow us to be absolutely sure of the circumstances of death, even if this results in unnecessary autopsies? The implications here are that, once again, medical truth is the best truth, and

---

[20] Collins, N. Changing Order: Replication and Induction in Scientific Practice. London: Sage (1985).

moreover, that the risk of not availing oneself of this incontrovertible information are too great for a coroner to take.

Such a belief in the truth and greater merit of the medical enterprise is demonstrated by pathologists in their response to family objections to coronial autopsy. Resentment is common when either the coroner or family objects to the undertaking of a three cavity internal autopsy. These take the form of suggesting that a partial internal autopsy should only be undertaken when only part of a body is available, and an increased suspicion and need to perform an internal autopsy when a family member raises an objection.[21] However, an over-reliance on autopsy as part of a coronial investigation, especially when other modes of enquiry may be open to the Coroner and pathologist,[22] have seen a large increase in objections to the forensic autopsy in Australia,[23] and a rise in the number of states in Australia and the USA which now include religious objections as an integral part of the coronial investigation.[24] The issue is that a thorough internal autopsy will almost always uncover information not otherwise discoverable. However, the question that remains is whether this is sufficient justification for the performance of internal autopsies in the coronial system?

3. WHAT VALUE IS ADDED BY AN INTERNAL AUTOPSY IN THE CORONIAL INVESTIGATION?

Given the increasing amount of evidence gathered at the scene of a death and thus available to coroners prior to their autopsy decision-making, it is possible to determine the accuracy of prediction as to cause of death prior to an autopsy being performed. For example, research supported by the Australian Research Council on Queensland coronial files in 2006 compared

---

[21] Barnes, M. "Reviewing reliance on internal autopsies". Address to the Asia Pacific Coroners Society Annual Conference. Auckland. (November 2010).
[22] Segal, G. "Law and Practice in relation to Coronial Postmortems – a social perspective". Medicine and Law. 25, 101-113. (2006)
[23] Lynch, M. "Forensic Pathology: Redefining Medico-Legal Death Investigation." Journal of Law and Medicine. 7 (August, 1999): 67-74; S. Emmett, S. Ibrahim, A. Charles and D. Ranson. "Coronial autopsies: a rising tide of objections." Medical Journal of Australia. 181, no.3 (2004): 173.
[24] Mittleman, R., Davis, J., Kasztl, W. and Graves, W. "Practical approach to Investigative Ethics and Religious Objections to the Autopsy." Journal of Forensic Sciences. 37, no.3 (1992): 824-829; Vines, P. "The Sacred and the Profane: The Role of Property Concepts in Disputes about Post Mortem Examinations." University of New South Wales Faculty of Law Research Series. Paper 13. (2007): http://law.bepress.com/unswwps/flrps/art13.

the cause of death deduced by non-medically trained researchers who considered only the information contained on the Form 1 - the initial report from police containing information immediately available at the scene - with that identified after autopsy. That process resulted in an error rate in accidental death of 8.4%, in suicide of 0.9% and in natural causes of 18.8%.[25] That level of accuracy sits within the accepted error rate of 30% of non-reportable deaths.[26], It is also likely that such error rates recorded by non-medical researchers would be significantly reduced in natural deaths most specifically, by a medical investigation before a decision as to whether an internal autopsy was necessary.

However, this high level of accuracy as to cause of death findings needs some clarification. In a number of situations, we determined that while detail was added by the autopsy, value to the coronial investigation was not. In these situations we suggested a high degree of predictive accuracy to the cause of death findings prior to autopsy. This may be challengeable in a medical or clinical respect, since detail and information was acquired during the autopsy. However, crucial to this discussion is whether or not such information added value to the cause of death finding and thus to the over-arching purpose of the autopsy in a coronial investigation.

For example, the blunt diagnosis "multiple injuries due to motor vehicle accident" dominated cause of death autopsy findings in accidental death, with 27.42% of all accidental deaths falling into this category. This was followed by "head injuries due to motor vehicle accident" which accounted for 19.05% of accidental deaths in the research timeframe. While in both cases, minor clarification was offered after the autopsy in some cases, we argue that this did not add any further detail to the cause of death finding than was apparent prior to autopsy in these cases. For example, rather than "multiple injuries due to MVA", findings after autopsy also included "head and chest injuries due to MVA", "massive soft tissue and bony trauma due to MVA", "chest and abdominal injuries due to MVA", and "multiple head/chest/abdominal injuries due to MVA". Similarly, rather than "head injuries due to MVA", findings after autopsy included "multiple fractures of skull due to MVA", "massive cerebral haemorrhage/trauma due to MVA", "intra-cranial haemorrhage due to MVA", and "cerebral contusions due to multiple fractures due to MVA".

---

[25] Carpenter, B., Barnes, M., Adkins, G., Naylor, C., Tait, G. and Begum, N. (2008) The coronial system in Queensland: the effects of new legislation on decision making. Journal of Law and Medicine, vol 16, no. 3, pp458-465.

[26] Burton J, Underwood J, (2007) "Clinical, educational and epidemiological value of autopsy", Lancet, vol 369, p1477

"PE due to DVT", "PE due to right atrial/cardiac thrombus", and "anoxia due to PE due to DVT". In these three cases, the dissection of the deceased during the autopsy did add further detail to the knowledge of how the deceased died. However, it is suggested that the detail gained in these cases did not add sufficient value to the cause of death certificate to warrant an internal autopsy in every case.

Perhaps more controversially, in a number of cases, while the autopsy did add clinical detail, the authors questioned whether it added significant value to the coronial investigation, especially in terms of findings as to cause of death. In a number of cases the authors ascertained a high predictive capacity for some natural deaths which, strictly speaking, may not be clinically accurate. For example, the prediction prior to autopsy of "coronary atherosclerosis", has been linked after autopsy with the cause of death, "aortic aneurysm due to atherosclerosis", including "haemorrhage due to ruptured aortic aneurysm", "massive soft tissue bleeding due to ruptured aortic aneurysm", and "hypovolaemic shock due to ruptured aortic aneurysm". In such situations we have determined a predictive capacity of 96.55% of cases. This is based on the medical relationship between aortic aneurysm and atherosclerosis and thus, while not clinically accurate, the finding after autopsy does not contradict cause of death predicted prior to autopsy. In such cases it is argued that allowing such predictions to be seen as accurate, adequately serves the purpose of the death investigation and the finding as to cause of death without the need for a full internal autopsy, given that in no case where an accurate relationship was identified did the finding after autopsy contradict the prediction prior to autopsy. While in many cases detail was added, this is precisely the point. Internal autopsies, especially those of between five and seven dissections, will always increase the detail of information as to cause of death. The question offered in its place is whether such procedures always add value to a coronial investigation.

This is especially the case since the vast majority of deaths in Queensland are not reported to the coroner. This means that in Queensland, 88% of deaths annually are not as accurately determined as those that reach the current coronial system. The importance of a death certificate detailing atherosclerosis, myocardial infarction or ischaemic heart disease becomes dubious, given that the rest of the population must be satisfied by a best guess from the medical profession. While others may conclude that this can only be rectified by performing autopsies for all deaths in Queensland, the current situation in England and Wales, which sees 45% of all deaths referred to the coroner, and the concomitant lack of personnel, resources and quality of post-

While in accidental death investigation full internal autopsies predominated (67.6% of all autopsies performed), they were more likely to occur in those cases where cause of death offered more detail. Those which determined a cause of death finding as "head injuries due to MVA" had a full internal autopsy performed in only 58% of cases, and "multiple injuries due to MVA" had a full internal autopsy conducted in 65% of cases. In contrast, "haemorrhage due to multiple injuries due to MVA" had a full internal autopsy conducted in 91% of cases and "exsanguination due to multiple injuries due to MVA" had a full internal autopsy conducted in 83% of cases. This demonstrates precisely the point. Internal autopsies will certainly discover more detail about the death under investigation. However, in these cases at least, the authors would argue that no further value was gained by performing an internal autopsy in terms of the finding as to cause of death.

Interestingly for this research, the largest number of external-only autopsies were performed in death by suicide at 16.05%. This is in comparison with accidental deaths which had external-only autopsies in 8.57% of deaths, and death by natural causes which had an external-only autopsy in 1.04% of deaths. This tends to confirm our argument that death by suicide is mostly identified by the evidence at the scene rather than in an internal autopsy. Nevertheless, internal autopsies predominated in death by suicide cases with internal autopsies performed in 83.95% of cases.

In death by natural causes, a large percentage of the deaths were attributed to the all-encompassing "coronary atherosclerosis" or "coronary artery disease" (21.8% overall). Given the small number of external-only autopsies performed in death by natural causes (1.04% of total autopsies), such blunt diagnoses were generally the result of a significant number of internal dissections of the deceased. In these cases it is questionable whether the cost or purpose of the coronial autopsy was achieved. However, in the majority of cases the autopsy did add varying levels of detail to the cause of death finding. The question as to whether such detail also added value to either the death investigation itself or the cause of death certificate is a far more controversial issue to explore in this category of death. In some cases, this was a fairly unproblematic exercise. The case of the prediction prior to autopsy of "myocardial infarction" was linked with findings after autopsy which included "myocardial infarction due to atherosclerosis", "myocardial infarction due to ischaemic heart disease", "acute cardiac failure/cardiac arrest", "acute coronary artery occlusion", and "cardiac tamponade due to acute myocardial infarction". Similarly, when the predicted cause of death was "pulmonary embolism" prior to autopsy, this was linked to findings after autopsy including mortem examinations,[27] indicates that such a system is neither sustainable nor desirable.

4. WHAT IS THE PURPOSE OF AN INTERNAL AUTOPSY IN A CORONIAL INVESTIGATION?

The question of the purpose of the Coronial autopsy is an extremely important one in the context of this discussion, and it is also the question which causes most confusion and uncertainty within the coronial system. In England, the 2004 *National Confidential Enquiry into Patient Outcome and Death* (NCEPOD) review of autopsy reports highlighted the fact that many Coroners themselves did not always seem to be clear on exactly what they were looking for in the post-mortems,[28] while Roberts et al (2000) reported in her survey of ninety one medical examiners, that pathologists themselves are divided over the role and purpose of the Coronial autopsy.[29]

Part of the problem is that terms like "cause of death", "manner of death" and "circumstance of death" are insufficiently precise to encompass a wide variation in practice and there has been little discussion to resolve the possible ambiguities. There can be no consensus about the level of autopsy required in a particular case unless these doubts are resolved. In Australia, Coroners Acts variously restate the traditional "manner and cause of death" as the "medical cause of death", "how the person died" or "the circumstances of the death".[30] No guidance is given as to the degree of certainty required or to the level of specificity with which the cause of death should be described. Both issues are crucial to a determination of the level of autopsy that is appropriate.

---

[27] United Kingdom, Constitutional Affairs Committee, Reform of the Coroners' System and Death Certification. Eighth Report of Session 2005-2006 (House of Commons, London, 2006) p 49.
[28] Ranson, D. (2007), Coroners' autopsies: quality concerns in the United Kingdom. Journal of Law and Medicine; 14: 315-318.
[29] Roberts, I., Nolte, K., Warner, T., McCarty, T., Rosenbaum, L. and Zumwalt, R. "Perceptions of the Ethical acceptability of using medical examiner autopsies for research and education." Archives of Pathology and Laboratory Medicine. 124, no.10 (2000): 1485-1495.
[30] See for example, Coroners Act 2006 (NZ) s57(2); the Coroners Act 1996 (WA) s25(1); the Coroners Act 2003 (Qld) s45(2)

a.) Natural Deaths

When deaths by natural causes are certified rather than reported to a coroner there is only a requirement that the probable cause of death be shown on the certificate.[31] As noted previously, the generally accepted error rate for such certificates when issued in hospitals is around 30%.[32] In Australia, only between 10% and 15% of all deaths are referred to a coroner for investigation – about half these are identified at the outset of being due to natural causes.[33] If the community is prepared to accept a 30% error rate in relation to the 90 – 95% of natural causes deaths that are not reported to the coroner, is it inconsistent to insist on certainty as a justification for the undertaking of internal autopsies in non suspicious, natural causes, reportable deaths. If the *probable* cause is sufficient certainty in the deaths that are certified without reference to a coroner, why should a higher standard be used to determine whether an autopsy is required for those that are?

It is also open to discussion whether an internal autopsy is justified to refine a finding of a natural cause that can be comfortably made without one. For example, who benefits from knowing an elderly individual died from a myocardial infarction rather than the more general ischemic heart disease? On the other hand, when an apparently healthy infant or young adult dies unexpectedly an internal autopsy will usually be warranted to establish the proximate cause of death and to ascertain whether other family members may be at risk of premature death.

Similarly, it is questionable whether a coroner is responsible for the accuracy or precision of mortality statistics. These aggregated data can be sought from hospital records and death registries. While accuracy is desirable, it is not clear that an internal autopsy is justified if the general cause of death is otherwise able to be identified, especially when a change in practice would impact on such a small percentage of the natural cause deaths – only 6.6% of all deaths are reportable natural cause deaths and only some of that number would be effected.[34] In any event, medical doctors routinely diagnose disease and prescribe treatment based on a clinical history, blood tests and non invasive procedures. Exploratory surgery is not routinely undertaken to exclude possibilities that have not been considered likely.

---

[31] Birth Deaths and Marriages Act 2003 s30(1)(b).(Qld)
[32] Burton J, Underwood J, (2007) opcit, p1477
[33] Barnes (2010) opcit,
[34] Queensland Office of the State Coroner, Annual Report 2009-2010. http://www.courts.qld.gov.au/1710.htm

b.) Unnatural Deaths

In many unnatural deaths the manner of death will be apparent from the scene and eye witness accounts. While in such cases an internal autopsy may yield more information, as with all other cases, consideration needs to be directed to the extra information necessary for the coroner's purposes to be achieved. This may best be illustrated by looking at a few common categories of unnatural deaths.

In theory, suspicious deaths do not necessarily and invariably require internal autopsies. However as suspicious deaths account for less than 2% of reported deaths[35] and as the consequences of compromising a homicide prosecution are so far reaching for those involved with the case and for the coronial system, it makes sense to accept that in almost all such cases an internal autopsy should be undertaken. That does not mean however, that all external causes deaths should have a three cavity autopsy to exclude the possibility of homicide. In most cases the likelihood of homicide is apparent at the outset. In cases where it is not, an internal autopsy may certainly be necessary, but only if another cause and manner of death cannot be established to the requisite standard.[36]

Internal autopsies can play an important part in establishing the manner of death. Identifying hidden homicides has always been central to the role of the coroner and pathologists have greatly assisted with this. If, however, wrongful third party involvement can be confidently excluded by other evidence and there is no other reason to undertake an internal autopsy, it is not clear that an internal autopsy should be undertaken "just in case." In all coroners cases further inquiries could almost always be undertaken but at some point the coroner assesses the available evidence as being sufficient to enable the necessary findings to be made. For example, whenever an inquest is conducted, information is discovered that was previously unknown. That does not lead coroners to conclude that all cases should go to inquest.

In most types of unnatural death investigations greater reliance on scene, eye witness and circumstantial evidence can frequently obviate the need for internal autopsies.[37] However, for the reasons discussed earlier, pathologists seem unwilling to place the same reliance on evidence sourced external to the

---

[35] ibid
[36] Davidson, A., McFarlane, J. and Clark, J. Differences in Forensic practice between Scotland and England. Medicine, Science and the Law, (1998), 38(4), 283-288.
[37] Pounder, D., Jones, M and Peschl, H. 'How can we reduce the Number of Coroners' Autopsies?: lessons from Scotland and the Dundee Initiative". Unpublished paper. (2009)

body. Some take an unduly reductionist position and claim they cannot exclude what they have not looked for notwithstanding the weight of the external evidence.[38] In many cases, further investigation could sufficiently establish the manner and cause of death without an internal autopsy. The body should be held while statements are urgently taken from the eye witnesses and an external examination and toxicology can confirm no third party involvement. Similarly, it is questionable whether an internal autopsy needs to be undertaken on all motor vehicle crash victims. Unexplained crashes by older drivers may warrant internal examinations to look for evidence of strokes or ruptured aneurysms. However, when an apparently healthy young person dies after a high speed crash little is to be gained, even less so in the case of passengers. Certainly nothing new is learned from reading an autopsy report which suggests "multiple injuries – mva" as the 1(a) cause of death, that could not be gleaned from the initial police report.

The biggest category of unnatural deaths reported to coroners are apparent suicides. An internal autopsy will rarely assist in distinguishing between a suicide, an accident and a homicide. Intent is the key element in suicide findings. It is usually to be inferred from notes or phone messages, previous attempts, triggering events and/or the circumstances of the death. While not suggesting that an internal autopsy would never be warranted, it is sensible to consider all of the other available evidence first. This was made starkly apparent by a recent murder trial concerning a jail hanging. A pathologist had attended the scene and a full internal autopsy was undertaken. A finding of suicide was made. Only when a prisoner who had been in the jail at the time "found God" did he confess to his involvement in the murder.[39] It has also been suggested that an internal autopsy can discover an organic brain disorder that can explain a suicide, reducing the distress of the family. In Queensland since 2003, the investigation of 4000 suicides has never revealed this outcome through internal autopsy.[40]

c.) Prevention

The legislation governing coroners in Australia and New Zealand require or invite a coroner investigating a death to consider whether it could be prevented and most also encourage attention to the possibility to

---

[38] Barnes 2010 opcit, n23
[39] Barnes (2010) opcit, n23
[40] ibid

improvements generally in public health and safety in circumstances related to or connected with those in which the death occurred.[41] Comments or recommendations aimed at reducing risk or effecting other improvements can be included in the coroner's report.

It would be possible to use this aspect of a coroner's jurisdiction to justify the extensive use of internal autopsies. For example, undertaking internal autopsies in all natural causes deaths and publishing the reports in relation to any unusual findings could contribute to the creation of new knowledge concerning the pathology of disease. Alternatively, providing a copy of the report to a deceased patient's treating doctors would in many cases increase their understanding of the disease processes that led to the death, making them more knowledgeable doctors and thus save the lives of future patients. Taking this line of reasoning to its logical conclusions, conducting autopsies on all reportable deaths would lead to the creation of a longitudinal data set that is likely to provide a rich lode for multiple research projects, some of which at least, would contribute to improvements in public health and medical practice.

There are a number of problems with this approach. First, in practice unusual autopsy results are rarely written up and published. Second, even though coronial offices create procedures to ensure treating clinicians can easily get access to autopsy reports, they avail themselves of it rarely.[42] In the vast majority of cases autopsy reports simply lie on the file. And third, higher courts have held the prevention function is ancillary and subsidiary to the primary function. This means a coroner can only make inquiries to support findings on the manner and cause of death and cannot make inquiries simply to lay a foundation for preventative recommendations.[43]

Another focus of internal autopsies that could arguably come within the prevention justification relates to the detection of inheritable diseases or conditions. Indeed some pathologists have gone so far as to suggest pathologists owe a duty of care to family members to detect and report these conditions.[44] While the practice in Queensland is to willingly make any material gathered during autopsy available to family members for the investigation of such conditions, it is not clear that such information should influence the decision as to the extent of the autopsy.[45] In cases that might

---

[41] For example see the Coroners Act 2003 (Qld) s3(d) and s46; the Coroners Act 2006 (NZ) s3(1)(b) and s57(3); the Coroners Act 1996 (WA) s25)(2)
[42] Barnes 2010 opcit, n23
[43] Harmsworth v The State Coroner [1989] VR 989
[44] Ong, B. and Milne, N. (2007) "Limited post-mortem examination. An alternative and viable way to avoid full examination?" Forensic Science and Medical Pathology. 3, p188-193
[45] Barnes 2010 opcit n23

involve such considerations the circumstances of the death are likely to mean that an internal autopsy will usually be undertaken, for example, the sudden death of an apparently healthy teenager. In those cases an indication that the death may have been caused by a genetic condition is relevant to the cause of death and would of course be shared with the family and tissue made available to search for relevant gene markers. However, that does not suggest that coroners should be ordering internal autopsies in cases where findings as to manner and cause of death could be made without such an examination, solely to look for or exclude such information.

As a case in point, there are three fulltime coroners in Brisbane and they have been actively trying to ensure that the autopsy ordered is no more invasive than is necessary for the case in question. In 2009-2010, these three full time coroners ordered a full internal autopsy in 57% of reported deaths, and an external only autopsy in 20.8% of reported deaths. The results of this approach can be contrasted with the rest of the state where part time coroners and less experienced full time coroners are less inclined to resist pathologists' urging to order full internal autopsies, and as a consequence ordered internal autopsies in 79.29% of deaths, and external only autopsies in 7.5% of deaths. Comparison with other jurisdictions is difficult because of different criteria for reporting deaths to coroners. However, a data set from Dundee Scotland where the chief forensic pathologist has views similar to those expressed in this chapter shows remarkable trends in the reduction of internal autopsies, with external autopsies increased from 15% to 50% of cases between 1988 and 2007.[46]

With close attention to the medical records of the deceased and regard to the clinical symptoms witnessed by those with the deceased in the minutes or hours immediately before the death, the probable cause of death could be ascertained without autopsy in many cases. And indeed this is happening already in Australia, with an increasing number of cause of death certificates being issued by the pathologists who in consultation with the coroner review the deceased person's records and the results of a CT scan before an autopsy order is made.[47]

---

[46] Pounder etal (2009) opcit n49
[47] Clark, M. J. "Autopsy", The Lancet, 366, p1767 (2005)

Conclusion

In England, Wales, Australia and New Zealand unnecessary internal autopsies are being undertaken. Unnecessary in the sense that they are not required to discover information the investigating coroner needs to make the required findings. This is happening because of the different traditions and epistemologies of coroners and pathologists and a lack of consensus about what coronial investigations should be seeking to establish. Pathologists place greater weight on scientific evidence they can source from the body at autopsy. They have much less regard for the evidence, opinions and views of witness or family members. They strive for scientific certainty whenever possible. Some pathologists believe they can not reach a conclusion about likely cause of death without conducting a three cavity autopsy because many of their conclusions are diagnoses of exclusion.

The point here is not to marginalise forensic pathologists in the coronial jurisdiction. Rather, it is to suggest that their expertise could be better deployed by more intensively reviewing case material before a decision as to whether an internal autopsy is needed, is made by the coroner. This approach has been adopted in Melbourne, Australia and it has resulted in a steep decline in the number of internal autopsies.[48] Currently, in Queensland and other Australian jurisdictions, the focus is on releasing the body as soon as possible.[49] However, if gathering more information in the days after the death means an unnecessary internal autopsy can be avoided, the delay occasioned by making those inquiries is justified. Such an approach would help redress another more serious delay, namely that encountered when obtaining autopsy reports. Last year in Queensland, 55% of those reports were received within a 3 months but 20% took more than 6 months. Reducing the number of autopsies undertaken is likely to mean most reports are received more quickly.[50] It would also enable pathologists to devote more time to intensively investigating other matters. In particular, their expertise in reviewing hospital deaths would be of great assistance to coroners.[51] Coroners and pathologists need to engage in more discussion about what it is coroners and bereaved

---

[48] Victorian Office of the State Coroner, Annual Report 2008-2009. http://www.coronerscourt.vic.gov.au/
[49] Barnes 2010 opcit,
[50] Qld Office of the State Coroner, opcit,
[51] It has previously been recommended that the Office of the State Coroner be funded to engage a fulltime medical officer to advise coroners in relation to such matters – see Queensland Hospitals Public Commission of Inquiry Report, 2005, p536. http://www.qphci.qld.gov.au . However, this has not occurred and so forensic pathologists are a valuable resource.

families actually need from coronial investigations. This conversation would give greater precision to terms such as manner and cause of death.

In: Pathology: New Research
Editors: J. M. Vultagione et al.
ISBN: 978-1-62100-698-5
© 2012 Nova Science Publishers, Inc.

Chapter 3

PSYCHOPATHOLOGY OF SUICIDE IN BALI

Toshiyuki Kurihara[*1] *and Motoichiro Kato*[‡2]

[1]Department of Psychiatry, Komagino Hospital, Tokyo, Japan
[2]Department of Neuropsychiatry, Keio University School of Medicine, Shinjuku, Tokyo, Japan

ABSTRACT

Although suicide is one of the major causes of death worldwide, research regarding suicide in developing countries is still lacking. In this chapter, we discuss the psychopathology of suicide in Bali, Indonesia. In the first section, we present research investigating the suicide rate in Bali. An examination of case records from police stations and interviews with police, community leaders, doctors, and victims' families was conducted. This investigation revealed that the annual suicide rate in Bali was 4.6 per 100,000 population in 2006. In the second section, we describe a psychological autopsy study comparing 60 suicide cases and 120 living controls matched for age, sex, and area of residence. This study identified the following risk factors for suicide: at least one diagnosis of an Axis-I mental disorder, low level of religious involvement, and severe interpersonal problems. Overall, 80.0% of the suicide cases were

---

[*] Corresponding author: Department of Psychiatry, Komagino Hospital, 273 Uratakao, Hachioji, Tokyo 193-8505, Japan, Tel: +81-42-663-2222; Fax: +81-42-663-3286; E-mail: kurihara@sj8.so-net.ne.jp
[‡] Department of Neuropsychiatry, Keio University School of Medicine, 35 Shinanomachi, Shinjuku, Tokyo 160-8582, Japan, Tel: +81-3-3353-1211; Fax: +81-3-5379-0187; E-mail: motokato@tc4.so-net.ne.jp

diagnosed with mental disorders; however, only 16.7% had visited a primary care health professional and none had received psychiatric treatment during the 1 month prior to death. These results highlight the importance of early recognition and treatment of mental disorders, religious activities, and interpersonal problem-solving strategies for suicide prevention in Bali.

I. SUICIDE RATE IN BALI

1. Introduction

In the year 2000, approximately one million people died of suicide, which represents a global mortality rate of 16 per 100,000 or one death every 40 seconds (World Health Organization, 2011). According to the WHO report, suicide rates among young people have been increasing, and they are currently the group at highest risk in one third of all countries where suicide data are available. There is rising concern for the attendant pain, societal disruption, and economic drain caused by suicides (Hoven et al., 2010). Despite the fact that suicide is a major public health problem worldwide, data on suicide rate are unavailable for 73% of developing countries, including Indonesia. In Bali, one of the Indonesian islands, Suryani et al. (2009) demonstrated that the suicide rate in the period following the 2002 Bali bombings was 8.10 for males and 3.68 for females per 100,000 population. However, they investigated the suicide rate in only three of nine administrative regencies in Bali, and did not indicate the overall year-by-year suicide rate of the targeted population. The present study aimed to investigate the suicide rate in all nine regencies in Bali in 2006. The study was approved by the Indonesian Institute of Science.

2. Methods

2.1. Study Area

Bali is one of more than 15,000 islands that make up Indonesia, which is categorized among the lower-middle income countries (World Bank 2011). In 2006, Bali's population was 3,263,296, and the island is almost entirely ethnically and culturally homogeneous. While Bali is famous as a tourist resort, most Balinese people engage in primary industries. An extended family system is common in Bali, and the basic unit of society is a community referred to as a *banjar*, consisting of up to several hundred households. Most Balinese consider the religious and social activities of the *banjar* to be essential parts of their lives. In 2006, Bali had 310 psychiatric beds, and the number of psychiatric beds per 10,000 population was low (1.0).

2.2. Data Extraction

Suicides were extracted from case records for the period between January and December 2006 from 53 police stations accounting for the entire population of Bali. For each suicide, the first author (T.K.) collected information regarding the conditions of death from police, community leaders, doctors, and the victims' families. After all information was thoroughly reviewed by the research team, the cause of death in all cases was determined to be suicide. The entire population count and population estimates by age group in 2006 were based on census data (BPS- Statistics of Bali Province, 2007).

3. Results

We identified 149 suicides in 2006. The overall, male, and female suicide rates in 2006 were 4.6, 6.1, and 3.0 per 100,000 people, respectively. Suicide rates per 100,000 population by age groups were as follows: 10 - 14, 0.8; 15 - 24, 6.5; 25 - 34, 4.2; 35 - 44, 3.7; 45 - 54, 5.0; 55 - 64, 6.6; 65 - 74, 11.6; >74, 15.7. One hundred and seventeen (78.5%) of the 149 suicides died by hanging, 23 (15.4%) by poisoning, 4 (2.7%) by stabbing, 2 (1.3%) by drowning, 2 (1.3%) by jumping from a height, and 1 (0.7%) by burning.

4. Discussion

To our knowledge, this is the first successful study examining the annual suicide rate of the entire population of Bali. The suicide rate found in the present study was slightly lower than that found by Suryani et al. (2009) and markedly lower than the world average. However, suicide remains a critical public concern in Bali, as the suicide rate has significantly increased (nearly four-fold in males and three-fold in females) since the 2002 bombings of three of nine administrative regencies in Bali (Suryani et al., 2009). Now is an appropriate time for health professionals to recognize suicide as a major health problem and focus on suicide prevention.

Suicide rate was higher among older people. Males were approximately twice as likely to commit suicide as females; this tendency is similar that observed in developed countries, but not other developing countries in Asia. In China, for example, female suicides are 25% more common than male suicides (Phillips et al., 2002a), and in India, female adolescents are more than twice as likely as male adolescents to commit suicide (Aaron et al., 2004).

This study has several limitations. The suicide rate reported in this study may be underestimated due to underreporting in areas where, because suicide is still considered a taboo topic, people might try to conceal the cause of death of relatives. An inadequate registration system or families' efforts to avoid police investigation may also contribute to underestimation of the suicide rate. Despite this limitation, however, we believe that this study represents an initial step for further research attempting to determine more accurate estimates of the suicide rate in Bali. Future study should employ verbal autopsy methodology similar to the study conducted in south India (Gajalakshmi and Peto, 2007), in which an epidemiological survey was carried out to identify all deaths in the target area and field interviewers determined the cause of death.

II. RISK FACTORS FOR SUICIDE IN BALI: A PSYCHOLOGICAL AUTOPSY STUDY

1. Introduction

Although the suicide rate in Bali was lower than the world average, as described in the previous section, the finding that the suicide rate has significantly increased in recent years suggests that suicide should be recognized as a major health problem. Given that suicide rate is probably underestimated due to underreporting of suicides, the actual impact of suicide on mortality in Bali is most likely much higher. Moreover, as the Balinese Hindu religion considers suicide to be an offense against the gods that leads to punishment in the next life (Jensen and Suryani, 1992), suicide is a major social concern in Bali. Another important reason why suicide is a major public health problem is its effect on the lives of victims' families, friends, and intimate community members. Friends and family members of people who have committed suicide experience more severe health consequences and grief reactions than those who have been bereaved through other causes of death (Ness and Pfeffer, 1990). Suicide bereavement is distinct in three significant ways: the thematic content of the grief, the social processes surrounding the bereaved individual, and the impact on family systems (Jordan, 2008). Not being prepared for the death carries a high likelihood of complicated grief for the bereaved, and if the death was violent, it is often associated with the onset of major depression (Barry et al., 2002; Sakinofsky, 2007).

There are a range of factors associated with suicide related to distal causes (such as social position, economic factors, social isolation and integration, and cultural factors) and more proximate causes (such as psychiatric illness, personality, psychobiological factors) along a hypothetical etiological pathway to suicide (Maris, 2002; Li et al., 2011). To our knowledge, however, no study has been conducted in Bali examining risk factors for suicide. Although studies from other Asian countries have demonstrated that risk factors for suicide are similar to those in western countries (Vijayakumar and Rajkumar, 1999; Cheng et al., 2000; Phillips et al., 2002b; Chiu et al., 2004; Zhang et al., 2004; Chen et al., 2004; Li et al., 2008; Khan et al., 2008; Wong et al., 2008) culturally or socially unique findings are also noted in each study. For instance, Phillips et al. (2002b) showed that the presence of a psychiatric disorder was not a significant predictor of suicide in the final regression model in China, although a substantial amount of published work from western countries has reported a link between psychiatric disorders and suicidal behaviors. Moreover, Chen et al. (2004) demonstrated that socio-economic adversities such as unemployment and debt have played an important role in suicide in Hong Kong during the recent economic recession. Therefore, in order to establish a culturally appropriate suicide prevention program, it is essential to investigate the risk factors for suicide that are particular to each region. The psychological autopsy method, which is based on interviews with informants close to the deceased, is currently the most direct technique to examine the relationship between specific factors and suicide (Cavanagh et al., 2003).

The aim of the present study is to examine socio-demographic, clinical, and psychosocial correlates for suicide in Bali using a case-control psychological autopsy approach. This is the first study to investigate risk factors for suicide in Bali.

2. Methods

2.1. Participants

Sixty-four consecutive suicide cases were extracted from case records for a 4-month period in 2007 from all 53 police districts in Bali. The exact months of death were concealed to protect the identity of each case. The first author (T.K.) collected information regarding the circumstances of death from police, community leaders, doctors, and victims' families. After thoroughly reviewing all relevant information, the research team determined the cause of death to be suicide in all cases. Of the 64 extracted suicide cases, the families of 60 individuals (93.8%) participated in the study. The families of two cases refused to be interviewed. The remaining two families consented to participate in the study; however, they were unable to complete their interviews due to serious emotional distress. These two families were advised to seek appropriate psychiatric help immediately.

For each of the 60 suicide cases, two age- and sex-matched living controls were randomly recruited in the same village. The families of all the controls agreed to participate in the study.

The study was approved by the Ethics Committee of the Indonesian Institute of Science, and all participants gave written informed consent to participate.

2.2. Psychological Autopsy Interview

For each of the suicide cases and controls, two family members who were most familiar with the individual were chosen as the key informants. Although some subjects lived alone, many relatives lived in the same compound or neighborhood, as an extended family system is common in Bali. The first author (T.K.) conducted face-to-face interviews with all key informants (for both suicide cases and controls) in their homes. Psychological autopsy interviews (for informants of suicide cases) and interviews with informants of controls consisted of the same questions; however, the index date for controls was the date of interview, while it was the date of death for suicide cases. For the informants of suicide cases, the interview was performed between 3 and 12 months (mean 7.3 months; SD 2.82) after the victim's death. Each interview took approximately 2 - 3 hours for families of suicide victims and 1 - 1.5 hours for families of controls.

2.2.1. Socio-Demographic Data

The following data were collected: number of family members, marital status, history of divorce, educational status, history of migration, and work status. While many relatives live in the same compound or neighborhood in Bali, only the number of family members living under the same roof was counted in this study.

2.2.2. Negative Life Events

Negative life events that occurred in the 1 year prior to death were assessed using a checklist based on The List of Threatening Experiences (Brugha et al., 1985). Negative life events were classified into the following eight categories: severe interpersonal problems, severe work-related problems, serious physical illness, severe school-related problems, severe financial problems, serious illness of a family member, death of a close friend or family member, and severe problems with the police. The duration and impact of each negative life event on each individual were recorded.

2.2.3. Mental Health Factors

A structured clinical interview for DSM-IV Axis I disorders (SCID-I) (First et al., 1996) was used to establish the best-estimate current DSM-IV diagnosis over the 1 month prior to death (American Psychiatric Association, 1987). In this study, axis-I diagnosis included major depressive episode, schizophrenia and other psychotic disorders, substance-related disorders, anxiety disorders, and adjustment disorders. SCID has been translated and back-translated and has proved to be a reliable screening instrument for individuals with schizophrenia in Bali (Kurihara et al., 2005). In this study, for the purpose of accurate diagnosis of depression, we added culturally sensitive terms (e.g., "ngekoh", a frequently used word that means having low energy, no volition, or no will to communicate) to SCID. A similar technique was also employed in a psychological autopsy study in China, as the direct translation of depression is not frequently used in everyday Chinese (Phillips et al., 2002b; Philllips et al., 2007). In addition to psychiatric diagnosis, help-seeking behaviors for psychological problems both over the 1 month prior to death and throughout the individual's lifetime (i.e., seeking psychiatric treatment from mental health professionals, primary health care professionals, or traditional healers) and history of prescriptions for psychiatric medication were also recorded. Medical records were examined to obtain accurate information regarding diagnosis and treatment history whenever available.

2.2.4. Psychosocial Factors

The following data were collected: previous suicide attempts, family history of suicide, religious activities, and social support.

Religious activities were investigated as follows. Each village in Bali has three temples, and temple anniversary rituals are conducted three times every Balinese calendar year (210 days), each lasting for several days. Participation in these rituals—some of the most important ceremonies conducted in Bali—was used as a standard to gauge individuals' level of religious activity. Individuals who had not participated in any anniversary rituals during the 1 Balinese calendar year prior to death were considered to have a low level of religious activity.

Social support was examined using two modified subscales of the Duke Social Support Index (Landerman et al., 1989). For the assessment of subjects' size of social network, informants were asked whether the subjects had more than two non-family members in the area (within 1 hour) on whom they could depend or with whom they were very close. For the evaluation of subjects' frequency of social contact, informants were asked whether the subjects spent a significant amount of time with someone who did not live with them more than two times a week, on average, in the 1 month prior to death.

2.2.5. Coding Procedure

Two raters (R.R. and I.T), who were blind to the case-control status, made a psychiatric diagnosis of each subject independently based on the SCID-I interviews. Subjects' negative life events, mental health factors, and psychosocial factors were then coded. After the two raters' psychiatric diagnosis and coding was completed, the first author and the two raters held a consensus meeting to reach a final decision on each item for all subjects, focusing in particular on the items for which the two raters' diagnosis or coding did not coincide and any vague information found in the case records.

2.3. Statistical Analysis

Statistical analysis was conducted using SPSS software version 11.5 (SPSS Inc, Chicago, IL, USA). Data were analyzed in a case-control design. First, *univariate* logistic regression analysis was performed to examine the individual effect of each factor on suicide. Odds ratios and their 95% confidence intervals were calculated. Significant variables were then entered into a multivariate logistic regression model, and a back-forward elimination method was employed to identify the most stable model.

3. Results

3.1. Description of Suicide Cases

Of the 60 suicide cases, 38 were males and 22 were females. Mean age was 41.4 (SD 21.5: range 13 - 87) Age distribution was as follows: <15, 2; 15 - 24, 17; 25 - 34, 10; 35 - 44, 5; 45 - 54, 8; 55 - 64, 6; 65 - 74, 6; >74, 6. Forty-one (68.3%) suicide victims died by hanging, 9 (15.0%) by poisoning, 4 (6.7%) by jumping from a height, 3 (5.0%) by drowning, 2 (3.3%) by stabbing, and 1 (1.7%) by burning.

3.2. Univariate Logistic Regression Analysis

Table 1 compares socio-demographic data, negative life events, mental health factors, and psychosocial factors between suicide cases and controls. Only significant variables are listed. Compared with controls, suicide cases were more likely to have a history of divorce, have less education, live alone, and be unemployed.

Table 1. Characteristics of suicide cases and controls

	Suicide cases (n = 60) n (percent)	Controls (n = 120) n (percent)	Odds ratio (95% CI)
Socio-demographic data			
History of divorce	7 (11.7%)	4 (3.3%)	3.83 (1.08-13.65)*
Low education (≤9 years)	49 (81.7%)	75 (62.5%)	2.67 (1.26-5.67)*
Living alone	5 (8.3%)	1 (0.8%)	10.82 (1.23-94.81)*
Unemployed	25 (41.7%)	20 (16.7%)	3.57 (1.77-7.21)***
Negative life events			
Severe interpersonal problems	26 (43.3%)	10 (8.3%)	8.41 (3.69-19.19)***
Severe financial problems	14 (23.3%)	12 (10.0%)	2.74 (1.18-6.38)*
Serious physical illness	14 (23.3%)	10 (8.3%)	3.35 (1.39-8.08)**
Mental health factors			
At least one psychiatric diagnosis	48 (80.0%)	18 (15.0%)	22.67 (10.11-50.80)***
Past psychiatric treatment	8 (13.3%)	2 (1.7%)	9.08 (1.86-44.22)**
Past treatment from traditional healer	11 (18.3%)	6 (5.0%)	4.27 (1.49-12.18)**
Psychosocial factors			
Low level of religious involvement	27 (45.0%)	6 (5.0%)	15.55 (5.92-40.83)***
Small social network	17 (28.3%)	4 (3.3%)	11.47 (3.65-35.99)***
Low frequency of social contact	13 (21.7%)	10 (8.3%)	3.04 (1.25-7.43)*
Previous suicide attempt	12 (20.0%)	2 (1.7%)	14.75 (3.18-68.40)**
Family history of suicide	10 (16.7%)	3 (2.5%)	7.80 (2.06-29.56)***

*p < 0.05 **p < 0.01 ***p < 0.001

Suicide cases tended to experience more negative life events (i.e., severe interpersonal problems, serious physical illness, and severe financial problems) compared with controls. Suicide victims experienced interpersonal problems with spouses (n = 12; 20.0%), a boy/girlfriend (n = 4; 6.7%), parents (n = 3; 5.0%), children (n = 3; 5.0%), friends (n = 3; 5.0%), and other relatives/persons (n = 8; 13.3%). Seven (26.9%) of 26 suicide cases who experienced severe interpersonal problems had conflicts with multiple persons.

Suicide cases showed a significantly higher prevalence of psychiatric disorders; of 60 suicide cases, 48 (80.0%) had at least one current diagnosis of Axis-I mental disorder. The most prevalent disorder was major depressive episode (n = 31; 51.7%), followed by schizophrenia and other psychotic disorders (n = 9; 15.0%; 6 schizophrenia, 1 schizophreniform disorder, 1 psychotic disorder due to epilepsy, 1 psychotic disorder due to auditory impairment), substance-related disorders (n = 4; 6.7%; 3 alcohol abuse and 1 other substance abuse), adjustment disorders (n = 4; 6.7%), and anxiety disorders (n = 2; 3.3%; social phobia). Of individuals who were diagnosed with mental disorders, two had dual diagnoses; namely, mood disorder co-morbid with substance-related disorder.

Suicide cases were more likely to receive both psychiatric treatment and treatment from traditional healers for psychological reasons in the past than controls. Eight (13.3%) had received psychiatric treatment in their lifetime; however, all had discontinued psychiatric treatment at the time of death. Of 48 suicide cases with mental disorders, 8 (16.7%) had visited a primary health care professional during the 1 month prior to death. Including visits to traditional healers, 12 (25.0%) sought help for their problems (4 at a medical facility, 4 at a traditional healer, and 4 at both) during the 1 month prior to death. However, none of the suicide cases received psychotropic medication.

As for psychosocial factors, suicide cases were more likely to show a low level of religious activity compared with controls. Moreover, suicide victims had a smaller social network and a lower frequency of social contact than controls. Furthermore, suicide cases were more likely than controls to have a history of previous suicide attempts and a family history of suicide.

3.3. Multivariate Logistic Regression Analysis

Multivariate analysis identified three independent significant factors, as shown in Table 2. The presence of at least one psychiatric diagnosis had the strongest effect, followed by low levels of religious involvement and severe interpersonal problems.

Table 2. Multivariate model of risk factors for suicide comparing suicide cases and controls

	Adjusted odds ratio (95% CI)
At least one psychiatric diagnosis	14.84 (6.12 - 35.94)***
Low level of religious involvement	7.24 (2.28 - 22.95)**
Severe interpersonal problems	3.86 (1.36 - 11.01)*

*$p < 0.05$ **$p < 0.01$ ***$p < 0.001$

4. Discussion

In the present study, a wide range of psychosocial and clinical factors that may be related to suicide in Bali were examined. This is the first successful psychological autopsy study in this developing country setting with a high participation rate for both suicide cases and controls, face-to-face direct interviews with key informants, and all informants consisting of close relatives rather than non-family members such as friends and visiting nurses. The results indicated that risk factors for suicide include at least one psychiatric diagnosis, a low level of religious involvement, and severe interpersonal problems.

Mental disorder was the most influential risk factor for suicide in Bali. Associations between mental disorder and suicide are often understood in the context of biopsychosocial stressors that may or may not incorporate contextual dimensions of individuals' lives, but also focus on immediate psychobiological sequelae associated with mental disorder relating to cognition, behavior and biological predisposition (Maris, 2002; Li et al., 2011). Robins et al. (1957) found that 93% of 109 patients brought to a general hospital immediately after a suicide attempt suffered from psychiatric disorders. According to a systematic review of psychological autopsy studies of suicide (Cavanagh et al., 2003), mental disorder was the most strongly associated variable of those that had been studied, and the median proportion of cases of mental disorder was 90% (range: 86 - 97%). The results of the present study are therefore consistent with previous psychological autopsy studies, although the percentage of mental disorders in this study was slightly lower (80%) than previously reported. Major depression was the most common diagnosis (51.7%) among suicide cases with mental disorders. This finding is consistent with those from other psychological autopsy studies (Cavanagh et al., 2003). Schizophrenia and other psychotic disorders were the second most common diagnosis (15.0%). Hor and Taylor (2010) indicated that important factors associated with schizophrenia suicides were young age, male gender, higher level of education, depressive symptoms, history of suicide attempts, active hallucinations and delusions, presence of insight, comorbid chronic physical illness, and family history of suicide; some of these were also identified by the univariate logistic regression analysis in the present study. On the other hand, alcohol abuse, another predominant mental disorder, was observed in only four suicide cases (6.7%). This finding is not consistent with most other studies except for one study from Pakistan (Khan et al., 2008), an Islamic country where alcohol is legally banned. Although alcohol is not prohibited by Balinese Hinduism, alcoholism is very rare in Bali, as drinking may cause one to lose his or her sense of geological orientation (e.g., the direction of the holy mountain of Gunung Agung, which represents the positive forces of universe (Thong et al., 1992)). Economic factors or the Balinese people's aversion to losing control of their emotions may also contribute to the low prevalence of alcoholism in Bali.

A low level of religious involvement was also found to be a significant risk factor for suicide in Bali. Analysis of religious affiliation among people who have committed suicide revealed that the highest rates are observed among atheists (Bertolote and Fleischmann, 2002). Previous studies in developed countries revealed that religious participation decreases the risk of both suicide completion (Nisbet et al., 2000; Duberstein et al., 2004) and suicide attempts (Blackmore et al., 2008; Rasic et al., 2009). Possible causes for this effect include the broader social network and increased instrumental support provided by frequent religious participation (Blackmore et al., 2008; Ellis and Smith, 1991). In Bali, religious ceremonies integrate individuals into the society and provide a forum for the exchange of informational, emotional and tangible social support among community members. In addition, as many religions—including Balinese Hinduism—strongly prohibit suicide, it follows that adherence to these religious doctrines would make followers less likely to attempt suicide (Blackmore et al., 2008; Ellis and Smith, 1991). Therefore, both social support and religious doctrine appear to contribute to the relationship between religious activities and suicide. The results of the present study showed that religion remained a significant item in the final multiple regression model, while social support items (i.e., size of social network and frequency of social contact) did not; however, it is premature to conclude that religion has a stronger effect on suicide than social support, as the social support items used in this study were not comprehensive. Further examination is needed to explore the relationship between religious involvement and suicide in Bali using more detailed social support criteria. To our knowledge, this is the first psychological autopsy study in an Asian developing country to indicate a significant association between religious activities and suicide completion.

Severe interpersonal problems were also identified as a risk factor for suicide in the present study. This finding is similar to those from Western countries (Appleby et al., 1999; Beautrais, 2001;Harwood et al., 2006) and Asian countries (Phillips et al., 2002b; Zhang et al., 2004; Li et al., 2008). Interpersonal problems were more directly related to suicide than other negative life events, such as financial problems, in this study. In general, Balinese live in communities with high population densities where frequent community activities create complicated interactions among families and community members. In such a social setting, severe interpersonal problems may reach a critical point and make an individual more likely to attempt suicide.

This study suggests several candidate prevention strategies for suicide in Bali. The strongest risk factor for suicide identified in the present study was mental disorder—48 (80.0%) suicide cases were diagnosed with mental disorders. However, only 16.7% of these cases contacted a primary health care professional, and none had received any psychiatric treatment during the 1 month prior to death. This finding is contrary to results from developed countries, where a majority of suicide cases had visited a primary care physician during the 1 month before death (Andersen et al., 2000; Luoma et al., 2002). In Bali, public education aimed at fostering help-seeking behaviors in individuals with mental disorders is essential for suicide prevention. In addition, education programs for primary care health professionals on the recognition and management of mental disorders are important, and the accessibility and availability of mental health care in Bali must be improved. However, Chen and Yip (2008) point out that increasing the number of psychiatric professionals may not directly translate into a decrease in suicide rate, as the suicide rate in Taiwan has increased three-fold in the past decade despite a 100% increase in the number of psychiatrists. They argue that a community-based method, rather than a psychiatric or clinical approach, is more relevant and cost-effective in Asian countries. Although the treatment of mental disorders in Bali is essential, such community-based prevention strategies also appear to be important. In the present study, a low level of religious activities and severe interpersonal relationship problems were also identified as significant risk factors. For the former, community-based intervention by religious leaders may be beneficial, while for the latter, consultation with either community leaders or traditional healers may be effective. For instance, religious leaders may be able to inquire about the absence of withdrawn individuals from religious ceremonies and offer the individuals or their families a religious solution, and community leaders could function as mediators of interpersonal conflicts within the community. Through those processes, religious and community leaders may be able to develop and reinforce social networks to support individuals at risk of committing suicide. In this study, hanging was the most common method used for suicide. Biddle et al. (2010) demonstrated that hanging is frequently adopted because it is relatively certain, quick, and unlikely to damage the body or leave a disturbing image for others, and is straightforward both in terms of access to materials and ease of implementation. Although the prevention of suicide by hanging is difficult, prevention strategies could focus on providing the general public with more accurate information about the process and consequences of hanging to counter perceptions of its rapidity, and to introduce awareness of the possibility of neurological impairment on survival (Biddle et al., 2010; Gunnel et al., 2005).

The present study has several limitations. First, the methodological problems inherent to psychological autopsy studies should be noted—the interviewer was not blind to suicide/control status, and the long duration between time of death and interview may have caused recall bias on the part of the informants. However, in the present study, a careful consensus meeting was held for the coding process of each factor in an attempt to minimize bias. Second, the present study's small sample size makes the interpretation of the results rather difficult. Third, data extracted from police reports may be a major source of bias due to the underreporting of suicides.

In summary, the present study identified at least one psychiatric diagnosis, a low level of religious involvement, and severe interpersonal problems as risk factors for suicide in Bali. Both clinical and community-based suicide prevention strategies are essential. Future studies should evaluate which aspects of prevention strategies are effective for establishing the most relevant suicide prevention program in Bali. In those studies, not only the quantitative research methodology used in this study but also a qualitative research methodology should be employed to improve the sensitivity and appropriateness of the study protocols.

COMPETING INTERESTS

The authors declare that they have no competing interests.

ACKNOWLEDGMENTS

The authors wish to thank all institutes and participants, especially those who lost loved ones to suicide.

REFERENCES

Aaron R, Joseph A, Abraham S, Muliyil J, George K, Prasad J, Minz S, Abraham VJ, Bose A. (2004) Suicides in young people in rural southern India. *Lancet*, 363, 1117-1118.

Andersen UA, Andersen M, Rosholm JU, Gram LF. (2000) Contacts to the health care system prior to suicide: a comprehensive analysis using registers for general and psychiatric hospital admissions, contacts to general practitioners and practicing specialists and drug prescriptions. *Acta Psychiatr Scand*, 102, 126-134.

American Psychiatric Association. (1987) *Diagnostic and Statistical Manual of Mental Disorders, 4th edn (DSM-IV)*. Washington, DC: APA.

Appleby L, Cooper J, Amos T, Faragher B. (1999) Psychological autopsy study of suicides by people aged under 35. *Br J Psychiatry*, 175, 168-174.

Barry LC, Kasl SV, Prigerson HG. (2002) Psychiatric disorders among bereaved persons: the role of perceived circumstances of death and preparedness for death. *Am J Geriatr Psychiatry*, 10, 447-457.

Beautrais A. (2001) Suicides and serious suicide attempts: two populations or one? *Psychol Med*, 31, 837-845.

Bertolote JM, Fleischmann A. (2002) A suicide and psychiatric diagnosis: a worldwide perspective. *World Psych*, 1, 181-185.

Biddle L, Donovan J, Owen-Smith A, Potokar J, Longson D, Hawton K, Kapur N, Gunnell D. (2010) Factors influencing the decision to use hanging as a method of suicide *Br J Psychiatry*, 197, 320-325.

Blackmore ER, Munce S, Weller I Zagorski B, Stansfeld SA, Stewart DE, Caine ED, Conwell Y. (2008) Psychosocial and clinical correlates of suicidal acts: results from a national population survey. *Br J Psychiatry*, 192, 279-284.

BPS- Statistics of Bali Province. Bali in Figures 2007. (2007) *BPS- Statistics of Bali Province*, Denpasar, Bali.

Brugha T, Bebbington P, Tennant C, Hurry J. (1985) The List of Threatening Experiences: a subset of 12 life event categories with considerable long-term contextual threat. *Psychol Med*, 15, 189-194.

Cavanagh JT, Carson AJ, Sharpe M, Lawrie SM. (2003) Psychological autopsy studies of suicide: a systematic review. *Psychol Med*, 33, 395-405.

Chen EY, Chan WS, Wong PW, Chan SS, Chan CL, Law YW, Beh PS, Chan KK, Cheng JW, Liu KY, Yip PS. (2004) Suicide in Hong Kong: a case-control psychological autopsy study. *Psychol Med*, 36, 815-825.

Chen YY, Yip PS. (2008) Rethinking suicide prevention in Asian countries. *Lancet*, 372, 1629-1630.

Cheng AT, Chen TH, Chen CC, Jenkins R. (2000) Psychosocial and psychiatric risk factors for suicide. Case-control psychological autopsy study. *Br J Psychiatry*, 177, 360-365.

Chiu HF, Yip PS, Chi I, Chan S, Tsoh J, Kwan CW, Li SF, Conwell Y, Caine E. (2004) Elderly suicide in Hong Kong – a case controlled psychological autopsy study. *Acta Psychiatr Scand*, 109, 299-305.

Duberstein PR, Conwell Y, Conner KR, Eberly S, Evinger JS, Caine ED. (2004) Poor social integration and suicide: fact or artifact? A case-control study. *Psychol Med*, 34, 1331-1337.

Ellis JB, Smith PC. (1991) Spiritual well-being, social desirability and reasons for living: Is there a connection? *Int J Soc Psychiatry*, 37, 57-63.

First MB, Spitzer RL, Gibbon M, Williams JBW. (1996) *Structured Clinical Interview for DSM-IV Axis I Disorders*. New York: Biometrics Research Department, Psychiatric Institute.

Gajalakshmi V, Peto R. (2007) Suicide rates in rural Tamil Nadu, South India *Int J Epidemiol*, 36, 203-207.

Gunnell D, Bennewith O, Hawton K, Simkin S, Kapur N. (2005) The epidemiology *Int J Epidemiol*, 34, 433-442.

Harwood DM, Hawton K, Hope T, Harriss L, Jacoby R. (2006) Life problems and physical illness as risk factors for suicide in older people: a descriptive and case-control study. *Psychol Med*, 36, 1265-1274.

Hoven CW, Mandell DJ, Bertolote JM. (2010) Prevention of mental ill-health *Eur Psychiatry*, 25, 252-256.

Jensen GD, Suryani LK. (1992) *The Balinese people. A reinvestigation of character.* New York: Oxford University Press.

Jordan JR. (2001) Is suicide *Suicide Life Threat Behav*, 31, 91-102.

Khan MM, Mahmud S, Karim MS, Zaman M, Prince M. (2008) Case-control study of suicide in Karachi, Pakistan. *Br J Psychiatry*, 193, 402-405.

Kurihara T, Kato M, Reverger R, Tirta IGR, Kashima H. (2005) Never-treated patients with schizophrenia in the developing country of Bali. *Schizophr Res*, 79, 307-313.

Landerman R, George LK, Campbell T, Blazer DG. (1989) Alternative models of the stress buffering hypothesis. *American Journal of Community Psychology*, 17, 625-642.

Li XY, Phillips MR, Zhang YP, Xu D, Yang GH. (2008) Risk factors for suicide in China's youth: a case-control study. *Psychol Med*, 38, 397-406.

Li Z, Page A, Martin G, Taylor R. (2011) Attributable risk *Soc Sci Med*, 72, 608-616.

Luoma JB, Martin CE, Pearson JL. (2002) Contact with mental health and primary care providers before suicide: a review of the evidence. *Am J Psychiatry,* 159, 909-916.

Maris RW. (2002) Suicide. *Lancet*, 360(9329), 319-326.

Ness DE, Pfeffer CR. (1990) Sequelae of bereavement resulting from suicide *Am J Psychiatry*, 147, 279-285.

Nisbet PA, Duberstein PR, Conwell Y, Seidlitz L. (2000) The effect of participation in religious activities on suicide versus natural death in adults 50 and older. *J Nerv Ment Dis*, 188, 543-546.

Phillips MR, Shen Q, Liu X, Pritzker S, Streiner D, Conner K, Yang G. (2007) Assessing depressive symptoms in persons who die of suicide in mainland China. *J Affect Dis*, 98, 73-82.

Phillips MR, Li X, Zhang Y. (2002a) Suicide rates in China, 1995-99. *Lancet,* 359, 835-840.

Phillips MR, Yang G, Zhang Y, Wang L, Ji H, Zhou M. (2002b) Risk factors for suicide in China: a national case-control psychological autopsy study. *Lancet*, 360, 1728-1736.

Rasic DT, Belic SL, Elias B, Katz LY, Enns M, Sareen J, Swampy Cree Suicide Prevention Team. (2009) Sprituality, religion, and suicidal behavior in a nationally representative sample. *J Affect Dis*, 114, 32-40.

Robins E, Schmidt EH, O'Neal P. (1957) Some interrelations of social factors and clinical diagnosis in attempted suicide: A study of 109 patients. *Am J Psychiatry*, 114, 221-231.

Sakinofsky I. (2007) The aftermath of suicide: managing survivors' bereavement. *Can J Psychiatry*, 52(6 Suppl 1), 129S-136S.

Suryani LK, Page A, Lesmana CB, Jennaway M, Basudewa ID, Taylor R. (2009) Suicide in paradise: aftermath of the Bali bombings. *Psychol Med* 39, 1317-1323.

Thong D, Carpenter B, Krippner S. (1992) *A Psychiatrist in Paradise: Treating mental illness in Bali*. Bangkok: White Lotus Co.

Vijayakumar L. (2004) Suicide prevention: the urgent need in developing countries. *World Psychiatr,* 3, 158-159.

Vijayakumar L, Rajkumar S. (1999) Are risk factors for suicide universal? A case-control study in India. *Acta Psychiatr Scand*, 99, 407-411.

World Bank. World Bank list of economies. *http://go.worldbank.org/K2CKM78CC0* : accessed May 2011.

World Health Organization. Suicide prevention (SUPRE). Available online at *http://www.who.int/mental_health*. Accessed May 2011.

Wong PW, Chan WS, Chen EY, Chan SS, Law YW, Yip PS. (2008) Suicide among adults aged 30-49: a psychological autopsy study in Hong Kong. *BMC Public Health*, 8, 147.

Zhang J, Conwell Y, Zhou L, Jiang C. (2004) Culture, risk factors and suicide in rural China: a psychological autopsy case control study. *Acta Psychiatr Scand*, 110, 430-437.

In: Pathology: New Research
Editors: J. M. Vultagione et al.
ISBN: 978-1-62100-698-5
© 2012 Nova Science Publishers, Inc.

Chapter 4

PATHOLOGICAL EXAMINATION OF INFLUENZA VIRUS–ASSOCIATED AND AUTOIMMUNE ENCEPHALITIS/ ENCEPHALOPATHY IN CHILDREN

Masaharu Hayashi[*1], *Yasuo Hachiya*[1] *and Akihisa Okumura*[2]

[1]Department of Brain Development and Neural Regeneration, Tokyo Metropolitan Institute of Medical Science, Tokyo, Japan
[2]Department of Pediatrics, Juntendo University School of Medicine, Tokyo, Japan

ABSTRACT

Despite advances in treatments with antibiotics and prophylaxis by vaccinations, influenza virus–associated encephalitis/encephalopathy tends to be intractable and may be a cause of mortality and severe sequelae in children. In order to clarify the pathogenesis of childhood-onset encephalitis/encephalopathy, we conducted pathological examinations of brain tissue sections of these patients. First, in this

---

[*] Corresponding author: E-mail: hayashi-ms@igakuken.or.jp; Tel. +81-3-6834-2334; Fax +81-3-5316-3150, Department of Brain Development and Neural Regeneration, Tokyo Metropolitan Institute of Medical Science, 2-1-6 Kamikitazawa, Setagaya-ku, Tokyo 156-8506, Japan

review, we summarize the neuropathological features of influenza virus–associated encephalitis/encephalopathy of patients in Japan and present data on the involvement of oxidative stress in acute necrotizing encephalopathy. Second, we review the significance of autoantibodies against the glutamate receptor, glutamic acid decarboxylase, and voltage-gated potassium channels in childhood-onset neurological disorders. Finally, we show our immunohistochemical data on antineuronal autoantibody screenings using patient sera on control brain sections. In Japan, the incidence of subacute and focal encephalitis/encephalopathy during which children repetitively develop episodes of psychological abnormalities, convulsions, and/or involuntary movements has increased. Immune-modulating treatments are effective, indicating the possible involvement of autoimmune mechanisms. We compared the immunohistochemical results using serum from patients in the acute disease phase with those using serum from patients in the convalescent phase and explored the presence or absence of immunoreactivity that was localized to the symptom-related brain area. In three-fifths of the subjects, symptom-related immunoreactivity was identified in the cerebral cortex, hippocampus, basal ganglia, and/or thalamus. This screening method was useful for investigating the pathogenesis of focal encephalitis/encephalopathy in children.

INTRODUCTION

Remarkable advances in treatments with antibiotics and prophylaxis by vaccinations have contributed to improvements in the prognosis of patients with bacterial meningitis and viral encephalitis. Nevertheless, patients with influenza virus–associated encephalitis/encephalopathy tend to show a fulminant clinical course and be resistant to medical treatments, which may lead to high mortality and severe sequelae in children [1, 2]. In adults, autoimmune encephalitis occurs independently or in association with cancers and collagen diseases [3]. Children also develop autoimmune encephalitis/encephalopathy [4], but the detailed clinical characteristics and disease mechanisms remain to be investigated. In order to clarify the pathogenesis of influenza virus–associated and autoimmune encephalitis/encephalopathy in children, we have performed various pathological examinations. Here, we summarize the data from our laboratory and review the literature findings.

PATHOLOGICAL FEATURES OF INFLUENZA VIRUS–ASSOCIATED ENCEPHALITIS/ENCEPHALOPATHY

Several hundred Japanese children are affected by a severe form of influenza virus–associated encephalitis/encephalopathy, which is characterized by a systemic cytokine storm and vasogenic brain edema [1, 2]. Severe cases, which are complicated by multiple organ failure and disseminated intravascular coagulation (DIC), have a high rate of mortality. Such encephalitis/encephalopathy includes several specific disease types, and 3 of these, Reye-like syndrome, hemorrhagic shock and encephalopathy syndrome (HSES), and acute necrotizing encephalopathy (ANE), occur frequently and require careful recognition by physicians. In this paper, we delineate the characteristics of these 3 disease types and present our experience with representative cases.

Patients with Reye-like syndrome show a rapid and fulminant clinical course that is frequently associated with severe liver failure, but not congenital metabolic errors [1]. The main neuropathological finding in these patients is massive brain edema without inflammatory cell infiltration. In blood vessels, including those outside the brain, microemboli and hyalinization were observed in small vessels, suggesting endothelial damage and/or dysfunction of the blood brain barrier (BBB). Takahashi et al. reported a severe decrease in the levels of immunoreactivity for laminin α2 in the blood vessels of a 2-year-old girl dying from influenza virus-induced encephalopathy, although vascular changes were not identified by routine histochemistry [5]. The authors speculated that the decreased expression of laminin α2 in the blood vessels may have reflected a selective malfunction in the BBB. Our autopsy case was a previously healthy 3-year-old girl who developed fever. One day later, she experienced sudden cardiorespiratory arrest, and a legally ordered autopsy was done. She had no family history of neuromuscular disorders and showed normal development. The cerebrum showed severe edema, although the brain weight was not assessed. There was no necrosis in either the thalamus or brainstem (Fig. 1A). The lenticulate nucleus showed mineral deposits. Despite the acute deposition of fat droplets in the liver, the absence of data suggesting congenital metabolic errors led to the probable diagnosis of Reye-like syndrome.

HSES, which was originally described in the United Kingdom, is associated with acute-onset encephalopathy, hemorrhagic shock, watery diarrhea, severe DIC, and renal and hepatic dysfunction [6]. Brain computed tomography (CT) and magnetic resonance imaging (MRI) scans of patients with HSES have demonstrated edema of the entire cerebral cortex and occasional intracranial hemorrhages. Our autopsy case was a 7-year-old girl who suffered from severe myoclonic epilepsy of infancy from the age of 1 year and lacked a family history of congenital metabolic errors. She had suffered from an influenza virus infection that was associated with status epilepticus, and she died suddenly of acute cardiorespiratory failure. Both lungs showed severe bronchiolitis, and many hemorrhagic foci were found in the mediastinum and peritoneum. The brain demonstrated severe edematous swelling and weighed 1,275 g at autopsy (Fig. 1B). Ischemic changes were observed in the neurons of the cerebral cortex. However, neither the thalamus nor the brainstem showed necrosis, which was consistent with previous reports [7]. A bleeding tendency in the liver and severe brain edema supported the diagnosis of HSES.

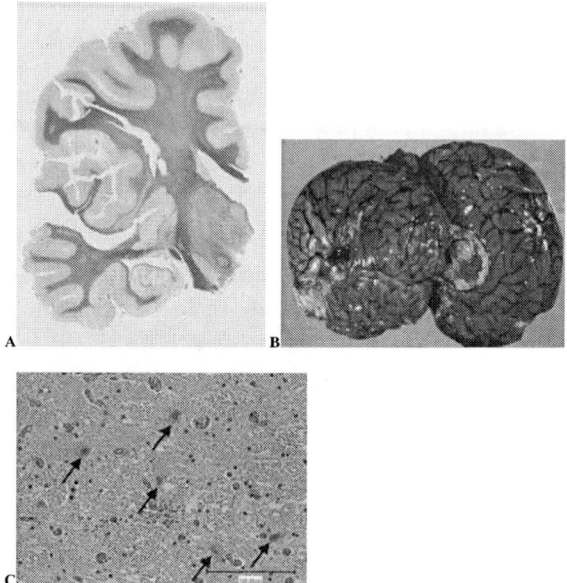

Figure 1. Neuropathological findings in patients with influenza virus–associated encephalitis/encephalopathy. A. The cerebral hemisphere demonstrated edema, and there was no necrosis in the thalamus in a 3-year-old patient with Reye-like syndrome, Klüver-Barrera staining. B. The cerebrum showed severe edema and subpial congestion in a 7-year-old case with hemorrhagic shock and encephalopathy syndrome. C. Neuronal sparing (arrows) was observed in the necrotic lesion in the pontine tegmentum in a 1-year-old case with acute necrotizing encephalitis, hematoxylin and eosin staining, bar = 100 μm.

ANE, which was first proposed in Japan [8], is prevalent in East Asia. ANE is characterized by diffuse brain edema and multiple focal lesions of necrosis and exudative vasculopathy, which are symmetrically distributed in both the thalami, the putamen, the cerebral and cerebellar white matter, and the brainstem tegmentum [9]. Our autopsy case was a 1-year-old boy, who had neither a family history of neuromuscular disorders nor infantile development abnormalities. He presented with a high fever. Two days later, he developed convulsions, a bleeding tendency, and liver dysfunction. He died of acute renal failure 1 day later. At autopsy, the brain was swollen and weighed 1,046 g, and necrotic lesions were found in both the thalami, the cerebellar white matter, and the brainstem tegmentum, as has been previously reported [10]. Adjacent to the necrotic lesions, there were microvacuolations, increased microvasculature, and neuronal sparing of the neuropil (Fig. 1C). Interestingly, these neuropil changes mimicked the pathological features found in mitochondrial myopathy, encephalopathy, lactic acidosis, and stroke-like episodes (MELAS) [11], which led us to conduct further immunehistochemical studies, as described below.

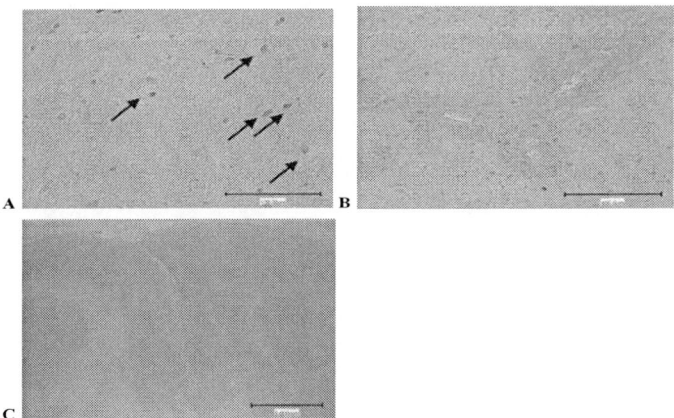

Figure 2. Immunohistochemical findings in patients with influenza virus–associated encephalitis/encephalopathy. A. Nuclei immunoreactive for 8-hydroxy-2′deoxyguanosine (arrows) were increased in the remaining neurons adjacent to the necrotic lesions in the thalamus in a 1-year-old case with acute necrotizing encephalitis, bar = 100 μm. B. Immunoreactivity for mitochondrial manganese superoxide dismutase was intensified around the vessels in the cerebral cortex in a 3-year-old case with Reye-like syndrome, bar = 400 μm. C.The levels of expression of excitatory amino acid transporter 1 were comparatively well preserved in the cerebral cortex of a 7-year-old case with hemorrhagic shock and encephalopathy syndrome, bar = 5 mm.

Pathological research conducted on autopsy brains can facilitate an understanding of the pathogenesis of cases of influenza virus–associated encephalitis/encephalopathy, but only a few of these studies have been done, partly because brain edema can prevent definitive staining in brain specimens. Nakai et al. investigated the presence of glial reactions and apoptosis in the brains of 8 cases of influenza virus–associated encephalopathy/ encephalopathy, including 2 with ANE [12]. The cases with probable Reye-like syndrome, but not the 2 with ANE, showed increased microglia, TUNEL-positive nuclei, and an increased expression of activated caspase-3, suggesting the involvement of microglial activation and apoptosis in Reye-like syndrome. We performed immunohistochemistry with markers for oxidative stress, antioxidant enzymes, BBB functions, and excitotoxicity in serial sections from the cerebral cortex, the hippocampus, the thalamus, and the brainstem, in cases of influenza virus associated with Reye-like syndrome, HSES, and ANE, compared to age-matched controls. We found nuclei immunoreactive for 8-hydroxy-2′deoxyguanosine (8-OHdG), a well-known oxidative stress marker of DNA, in the remaining neurons and glial cells adjacent to the necrotic lesions in a case of ANE (Fig. 2A). There were no changes consistent with facilitated lipid peroxidation. In addition, 2 ANE patients showed increased levels of 8-OHdG in the cerebrospinal fluid (CSF). In a 1-year-old girl with a chromosomal anomaly and a previously healthy 1-year-old girl, the CSF levels of 8-OHdG were 0.159 ng/mL and 0.129 ng/mL, respectively, surpassing the cutoff level (0.06 ng/mL). Adult MELAS patients showed increased levels of 8-OHdG in the CSF, and nuclei immunoreactive for 8-OHdG were found in perilesional surviving neurons in the cerebral cortex of autopsy cases of MELAS [13]. The spreading of lesions was prevented in some Japanese patients treated with edaravone, a medication involving radical scavengers that is approved for use in Japan. As aforementioned, cases of ANE and MELAS exhibited similar pathological changes in the neuropil. Taken together, it is possible that the oxidative stress of DNA may be involved in the neuropil changes in both disorders. Edaravone is used frequently in Japan for the treatment of patients with acute encephalitis/encephalopathy, including those that are influenza virus–associated, although a well-designed clinical trial of this medication has not yet been done. However, in a case of Reye-like syndrome, the levels of immunoreactivities for glial fibrillary acidic protein (GFAP), aquaporin 4 (AQP4), and manganese superoxide dismutase (MnSOD), a mitochondrial antioxidant enzyme, were significantly intensified around vessels in the cerebral cortex (Fig. 2B). Since the levels of GFAP and AQP4 in astrocytes modify the maintenance of BBB, the altered expressions of both molecules may suggest dysfunction of the BBB, similar to the abnormal expression of laminin α2 [5]. Furthermore, the expression of MnSOD is altered in mitochondrial disorders [14], and it is possible that mitochondrial impairment may be related to the BBB dysfunction in Reye-like syndrome. In contrast, the levels of excitatory amino acid transporters, which play a pivotal role in the prevention of excitotoxicity [15], were comparatively well preserved in cases of Reye-like syndrome, HSES, and ANE (Fig. 2C). The involvement of excitotoxicity in influenza virus–associated encephalitis/encephalopathy should be examined further in more cases.

PRESENCE OF ANTINEURONAL AUTOANTIBODIES IN CHILD NEUROLOGICAL DISORDERS

Rasmussen's encephalitis (RE) is a rare and progressive inflammatory disorder of undetermined etiology that occurs in children who characteristically present with refractory seizures, including epilepsia partialis continua (EPC), cognitive deterioration, and progressive hemiparesis [16]. The detection of autoantibodies against glutamate receptor (GluR) subunit 3 in RE patients suggested that an autoimmune process may be involved in the pathogenesis of RE [17]. The role of GluR3 in RE has been actively investigated, resulting in the accumulation of conflicting evidence on the pathogenic effect of GluR3 autoantibodies [18]. However, Takahashi et al. detected N-methyl-D-aspartate (NMDA)-type GluRε2 autoantibodies in the serum and/or CSF of patients with histologically proven and classical RE, encephalitis/encephalopathy, and EPC [19]. It is noteworthy that the onset of the EPC was in childhood in most of these patients. GluRε2 autoantibodies have been found in Japanese children with various neurological disorders, such as acute encephalitis with refractory and repetitive partial seizures [20] and enterovirus encephalitis [21]. GluRε2 autoantibodies were also detected in the CSF in adult patients with reversible autoimmune limbic encephalitis, whose symptoms were characterized by convulsions, psychiatric symptoms, and responsiveness to immunotherapy [22]. Since the levels of GluRε2 are associated with memory and learning [23], the autoantibodies against GluRε2 may contribute to the onset of mental deterioration in focal encephalitis. Recently, Dalmau et al. established a new category of treatment-responsive encephalitis that is associated with anti-NMDA receptor (NMDAR) antibodies, which are against the NR1/NR2 heteromers of the NMDAR [24].

Since Dalmau et al.'s review [25], which included an 11-year-old boy and 21 female patients younger than 19 years (median, 15 years; range, 5-18 years), the occurrence of NMDAR encephalitis is not uncommon in adolescents. Accordingly, 2 girls, who were aged 3 and 7 years, were reported to suffer from relapsing NMDAR encephalitis, in which neuropsychiatric disabilities persisted despite immune therapies [26]. Taken together, it is likely that autoantibodies against the NMDA receptor may cause autoimmune encephalitis/encephalopathy and modify the clinical course in children and adolescents.

Voltage-gated potassium channels (VGKC) are expressed in all tissues and contribute to the generation of cellular action potentials. VGKCs are potentially relevant to autoantigens in paraneoplastic syndromes [27]. Serum autoantibodies against VGKC have been reported in patients with epilepsy [28] and limbic encephalitis [29]. High titers of autoantibodies against glutamic acid decarboxylase (GAD) were originally detected in patients with stiff person syndrome [30]. In addition, they have been reported in patients with various neurological disorders, including cerebellar ataxia [31], nonparaneoplastic limbic encephalitis [32], and epilepsy [33]. It is not clear if these antineuronal autoantibodies are directly responsible for the neurologic manifestations in these patients. However, they may represent an underappreciated marker of immune-mediated neurologic disturbances. Accordingly, Sakuma et al. reviewed cases of Japanese children with acute nonparaneoplastic limbic encephalitis and stressed the possible involvement of infection-induced autoimmunity targeting neuronal antigens [4]. The examination of antineuronal autoantibodies should be considered in children with neurological disorders in which febrile illness that is presumed to be due to an infectious cause antecedes the neurological symptoms, the CSF suggests inflammatory changes, and immune-modulatory treatments are effective. Haberlandt et al. examined the presence or absence of specific neuronal autoantibodies in 10 patients aged less than 18 years who had clinicoradiologically proven limbic encephalitis [34]. Autoantibodies were observed in 8 patients. One patient with neuroblastoma demonstrated Hu antibodies, while 1 showed paraneoplastic syndrome-related Ma1/2 antibodies, and no tumors were found. Four patients revealed high titers of GAD antibodies, and 2 of these also had low titers of VGKC antibodies. Finally, only 2 patients had low titers of VGKC antibodies. These data strongly suggest that antineuronal autoantibodies against VGKC and GAD should be actively investigated in children and adolescents with limbic encephalitis.

IMMUNOHISTOCHEMISTRY WITH PATIENT SERA IN JAPANESE CHILDREN WITH SUBACUTE AND FOCAL ENCEPHALITIS/ENCEPHALOPATHY

In Japanese children, the incidence of subacute and focal encephalitis/encephalopathy during which patients repetitively suffer from episodes consisting of psychological abnormalities, convulsions, and/or involuntary movements has increased. Immune-modulating treatments, such as adrenocortical steroids and high doses of immunoglobulin, are effective, indicating the possible involvement of autoimmune mechanisms. However, the detection of autoantibodies against GluR/NMDAR, VGKC, and GAD is rare, and, therefore, the involvement of unknown antineuronal autoantibodies is speculated. Immunohistochemistry using patients' sera or CSF on human or animal brain sections has been employed in order to identify the antineuronal antibodies in cancer patients with paraneoplastic neurological syndromes [35]. The same method has been attempted in order to verify the presence of antineuronal autoantibodies in focal encephalitis involving the limbic system, the basal ganglia, and the cerebellum. In the aforementioned adult patients with reversible autoimmune limbic encephalitis in which autoantibodies against GluRε2 were detected the immunohistochemistry using patients' sera resulted in cytoplasmic immunoreactivity in neurons of the hippocampus and cerebral cortex [20]. Group A Streptococcus, which is the most common cause of pharyngitis, is a recognized cause of immune-mediated autoantibodies against neurons or glial cells in the basal ganglia. The classical phenotype, which is known as Sydenham's chorea and pediatric autoimmune neuropsychiatric disorders associated with streptococcal infections (PANDAS), has been proposed recently [36]. Antibasal ganglia antibodies have been identified with immunohistochemistry using the sera of patients with poststreptococcal autoimmune dystonia [37] and those with atypical dystonia and tics [38]. Furthermore, neuronal surface glycolytic enzymes were reported to be candidate autoantigens [39].

Table 1. Summary of immunohistochemistry using the patients's era

	Age/Sex	Category	Predisposing factor	Mental disturbances	Convulsion	Motor disability	Involuntary movements	Neuroradiological changes	Anti-neuronal antibodies	Immune-modulatory intervention	Prognosis	Immunoreactivity Cerebral cortex	Basal ganglia
Patients with positive immunoreactivity (PI)													
1	1yr/F	Focal encephalitis	(-)	1+	(-)	(-)	1+	Hypermetabolism on FDG-PET in the left cerebral cortex and basal ganglia	n/A	Steroid pulse, IVIG	Completely improved	Frontal and temporal cortex (Neurons)	Globus pallidus (Neurons)
2	3yrs/F	Basal ganglia encephalitis	Virus suspected	(-)	(-)	(-)	2+	T2-high signals on MRI in the left frontal white matter	n/A	Steroid pulse, IVIG	Persistent	(-)	Thalamus (Small neurons, Glial cells)
3	4yrs/F	ADEM	Vaccination	1+	1+	Paralysis	1+	T2-high signals on MRI in the basal ganglia and cerebral white matter	Glutamate receptor antibody	Steroid pulse, IVIG Cichosporin, anti-CD20	Remitted	Temporal and occipital cortex (Neurons)	Thalamus (Neurons)
4	6yrs/F	Basal ganglia encephalitis	(-)	1+	(-)	(-)	1+	Hypoperfusion on SPECT in the right basal ganglia	(-)	Steroid pulse	Completely improved	(-)	Putamen (Large neurons)
5	7yrs/F	PANDAS-like	Streptococcal	1+	(-)	(-)	(-)	(-)	Lysoganglioside antibody	IVIG	Completely improved	(-)	Globus pallidus (Neurons)
6	8yrs/M	Epileptic encephalopathy	Varicella virus	(-)	2+	Paralysis	(-)	T2-high signals on MRI in the right occipital and left occipital lobe	Lysoganglioside antibody	(-)	Remitted	Temporal and occipital cortex (Neurons)	(-)
7	9yrs/F	Focal encephalitis	Streptococcal	1+	(-)	(-)	(-)	(-)	Lysoganglioside antibody	Steroid pulse, IVIG	Remitted	Lateral occipitotemporal cortex (Neurons)	(-)
8	10yrs/F	ADEM	Streptococcal	1+	(-)	(-)	1+	T2-high signals on MRI in the bilateral basal ganglia	Lysoganglioside antibody	IVIG	Completely improved	(-)	Globus pallidus (Neurons)
9	13yrs/M	Limbic encephalitis	(-)	1+	1+	Paralysis	(-)	T2-high signals on MRI in the right temporal and insular cortex	n/A	Steroid pulse	Completely improved	Hippocampus (Neurons)	(-)
10	13yrs/F	Epileptic encephalopathy	Vaccination	1+	1+	Paralysis	(-)	Hypo- and hyperperfusion on SPECT in the right frontal and temporal cortex	Glutamate receptor antibody	Steroid pulse, IVIG	Remitted	Frontal cortex (Neurons)	(-)
Patients with absent immunoreactivity (AI)													
11	1yr/F	Focal encephalitis	Liver failure	1+	2+	Paralysis	2+	Mild volume reduction on CT and MRI in the frontal lobe	n/A	Steroid pulse	Remitted	(-)	(-)
12	1yr/M	Cerebellitis	RS virus	(-)	(-)	Ataxia	(-)	high signal in diffusion-weighted image on MRI in the cerebellum	n/A	Steroid pulse, IVIG	Persistent	(-)	(-)
13	1yr/M	Basal ganglia encephalitis	Virus suspected	1+	1+	(-)	1+	T2-high signals on MRI in the bilateral frontal and temporal cortex	Glutamate receptor antibody	Steroid pulse	Persistent	(-)	(-)
14	2yrs/M	Cerebellitis	Kawasaki disease	(-)	1+	Ataxia	(-)	(-)	n/A	IVIG	Completely improved	(-)	(-)
15	4yrs/F	Bilateral striatal necrosis	(-)	1+	(-)	(-)	1+	T2-high signals on MRI in the bilateral basal ganglia	n/A	Steroid pulse, IVIG	Persistent	(-)	(-)
16	11yrs/M	Limbic encephalitis	Virus suspected	1+	(-)	(-)	(-)	Hypoperfusion on SPECT in the bilateral frontal and temporal cortex	n/A	Steroid pulse	Completely improved	(-)	(-)
17	13yrs/F	ADEM	Streptococcal	1+	(-)	Paralysis	(-)	T2-high signal on MRI in the right basal ganglia and medulla	n/A	Steroid pulse, IVIG	Completely improved	(-)	(-)

Abbreviations are as follows: F, female; M, male; ADEM, acute disseminated encephalomyelitis; PANDAS, pediatric autoimmune neuropsychiatric disorders associated with streptococcal infections; RS, respiratory syncytial; FDG-PET, ^{18}F-fluorodeoxy-glucose-positron emission tomography; MRI, magnetic resonance imaging; SPECT, single photon emission tomography; CT, computed tomography; n/A, not assessed; Steroid pulse, treatment with high doses of methylprednisolone; IVIG, treatment with high doses of immunoglobulin.

In order to investigate the involvement of unknown antineuronal autoantibodies in Japanese children with the aforementioned focal encephalitis/encephalopathy, we performed immunohistochemistry on brain sections from age-matched controls without neurological disorders using the serum from patients in the acute disease phase and those in the convalescent phase (Table 1). If immunoreactivity was localized to the symptom-related brain areas and was only observed with the acute phase serum, it was speculated that the specific immunoglobulin in the patient serum bound to the neurons and/or glial cells in the symptom-related brain areas. We tested 17 subjects, and 10 patients aged 1 to 13 years (59%) demonstrated symptom-related immunoreactivity in the cerebral cortex, basal ganglia, and thalamus, whereas the other 7 patients aged 1 to 13 years (41%) did not. In patients 1 to 10 with positive immunoreactivity (PI) (Table 1), a female predominance (male:female = 2:8) was observed. Two patients each suffered from focal encephalitis, basal ganglia encephalitis, acute disseminated encephalomyelitis, and epileptic encephalopathy. For predisposing events, 3 and 2 patients experienced streptococcal infection and a vaccination just before disease onset, respectively. In patients 11 to 17 with absent immunoreactivity (AI) (Table 1), there was neither a sexual difference nor definite predisposing factors, although 2 patients had cerebellitis. There were no significant differences between the PI and AI patients in the occurrence of mental abnormalities, such as consciousness disturbances, excitement, obsessive compulsive disorders, and/or abnormal behaviors (PI, 70%; AI, 57%), convulsions (PI, 40%; AI, 43%), paralysis or ataxia (PI, 40%; AI, 57%), involuntary movements, such as dystonia, chorea, and tremor (PI, 50%; AI, 43%), or neuroradiological changes (PI, 80%; AI, 71%). Conventional antineuronal autoantibodies, such as antiGluR and antilysoganglioside antibodies, were detected in 5 of the 7 PI patients and 1 AI patients examined (Table 1). Most of the PI and AI patients received treatment with high doses of methylprednisolone, which was called steroid pulse therapy, and/or treatment with high doses of immunoglobulin, except for PI patient 6 with epileptic encephalopathy. The prognosis of PI patients (of the 10 patients, 5 completely recovered, and 4 remitted) was better than that of AI patients (of the 7 patients, 3 completely recovered, and 1 remitted). With immunohistochemistry, PI patient 1 showed neuronal immunoreactivity in the cerebral cortex and globus pallidus, corresponding to the patient's mental disturbances and involuntary movements, respectively, which was consistent with previous reports [40]. PI patients 2, 3, 4, and 8 with involuntary movements demonstrated immunoreactivity in neurons and/or glial cells in the globus pallidus, thalamus, or putamen (Fig. 3). In PI patient 5, the immunoreactivity observed in the globus pallidus may have been involved in the obsessive compulsive disorders mimicking PANDAS. In contrast, PI patients 6, 7, 9, and 10 demonstrated neuronal immunoreactivity in the cerebral cortex and/or hippocampus, corresponding to the patients' mental disturbances and/or convulsions.

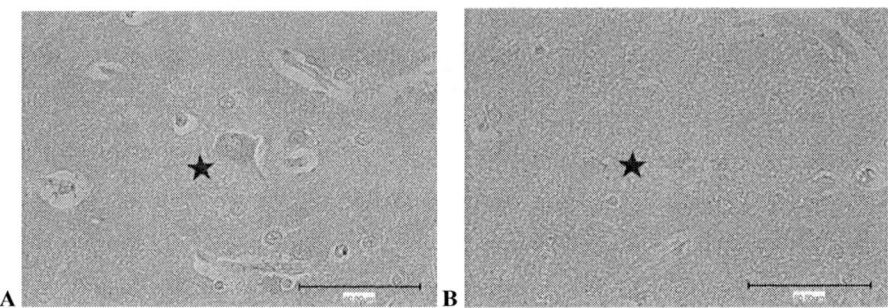

Figure 3. Immunohistochemistry in patient 4 with subacute and focal encephalitis/encephalopathy. A 6-year-old girl developed repetitive episodes that consisted of rapid exacerbation of chorea and ballismus from the age of 5 years and 1 month to 6 years and 1 month. Single photon emission computed tomography demonstrated hypoperfusion in the right basal ganglia. Treatment with high doses of methylprednisolone was effective in each episode, and symptoms were relieved gradually 2 to 4 weeks after the treatment. Tests for congenital metabolic errors and autoantibodies were all negative. The cytoplasm of large neurons (star) in the putamen in a control brain section exhibited immunoreactivity with the patient's serum at the acute phase (A), which was absent in those immunohistochemical sections using the serum of the patient at convalescence (B). Bars = 60 μm.

In conclusion, we believe that screening with immunohistochemical analyses is useful for exploring the pathogenesis of subacute and focal encephalitis/encephalopathy in children. Since the immunohistochemical results need to be confirmed by other methods [34], we are now preparing for future studies in which the brain antigens are restricted and the molecular weights of antigens are quantified using Western blotting. Recently, a new subtype of subacute encephalopathy in Japanese children was proposed [41]. The disease is characterized by onset of seizures, subsequent worsening of consciousness disturbances, mild cortical atrophy on late MRI scans, and poor neurologic outcomes. Immunohistochemical analyses using sera from these patients may also be useful for characterizing the pathogenesis of that disease, and we are planning an analysis in patients with such subacute encephalopathy.

REFERENCES

[1] Morishima, T; Togashi, T; Yokota, S; Okuno, Y; Miyazaki, C; Tashiro, M; Okabe, N; the Collaborative Study Group on Influenza-Associated Encephalopathy in Japan. Encephalitis and encephalopathy associated with an influenza epidemic in Japan. *Clinical Infectious Diseases* 2002, 35, 512-517.

[2] Mizuguchi, M; Yamanouchi, H; Ichiyama, T; Shiomi, M. Acute encephalopathy associated with influenza and other viral infections. *Acta Neurologica Scandinavica* 2007, 115(Suppl. 186), 45-56.

[3] Graus, F; Saiz, A; Dalmau, J. Antibodies and neuronal autoimmune disorders of the CNS. *Journal of Neurology* 2010, 257, 509-517.

[4] Sakuma, H; Sugai, K; Sasaki, M. Acute nonparaneoplastic limbic encephalitis in childhood: a case series in Japan. *Pediatric Neurology* 2010, 43, 167-172.

[5] Takahashi, M; Yamada, T; Nakashima, Y; Saikusa, H; Deguchi, M; Kida, H; Tashiro, M; Toyoda, T. Influenze virus-induced encephalopathy: clinicopathologic study of an autopsied case. *Pediatric International* 2000, 42, 204-214.

[6] Rinka, H; Yoshida, T; Kubota, T; Tsuruwa, M; Fuke, A; Yoshimoto, A; Kan, M; Miyazaki, D; Arimoto, H; Miyaichi, T; Kaji, A; Miyamoto, S; Kuki, I; Shiomi, M. Hemorrhagic shock and encephalopathy syndrome – the markers for an early HSES diagnosis. *BMC Pediatrics* 2008, 8, 43.

[7] Hayashi, M; Sugai, K; Kurihara, E; Tamagawa, K. An autopsy case of severe myoclonic epilepsy of infancy, who died of acute encephalopathy associated with influenza infection. *Epilepsia* 2004, 45(Suppl. 8), 65.

[8] Mizuguchi, M; Abe, J; Mikkaichi, K. Acute necrotizing encephalopathy of childhood: a new syndrome presenting with multifocal, symmetric brain lesions. *Journal of Neurology, Neurosurgery and Psychiatry* 1995, 58, 555-561.

[9] Ng, WF; Chiu, SC; Lam, DS; Wong, YC; Tan, S; Kwong, NS; Loo, KT; Yuen, KY. A 7-year-old boy dying of acute encephalopathy. *Brain Pathology* 2010, 20, 261-264.

[10] Nakano, I; Otsuki, N; Hasegawa, A. Acute stage neuropathology of infantile acute encephalopathy with thalamic involvement: widespread symmetrical fresh necrosis of the brain. *Neuropathology* 1993, 13, 315-325.

[11] Hayashi, M; Miyata, R; Tanuma, N. Oxidative stress in developmental brain disorders. In: Ahmad, SI, ed., *Neurodegenerative Diseases*, New York: Landes Bioscience and Springer Science, 2011 (in press).

[12] Nakai, Y; Itoh, M; Mizuguchi, M; Ozawa, H; Okazaki, E; Kobayashi, Y; Takahashi, M; Ohtani, K; Ogawa, A; Narita, M; Tagashi, T; Takashima, S. Apoptosis and microglial activation in influenza encephalopathy. *Acta Neuropathologica* 2003, 105, 233-239.

[13] Katayama, Y; Maeda, K; Iizuka, T; Hayashi, M; Hashizume, Y; Sanada, M; Kawai, H; Kashiwagi, A. Accumulation of oxidative stress around the stroke-like lesions of MELAS patients. *Mitochondrion* 2009, 9, 306-313.

[14] Hayashi, M; Araki, S; Kohyama, J; Shioda, K; Fukatsu, R. Oxidative nucleotide damage and superoxide dismutase expression in the brains of xeroderma pigmentosum group A and Cockayne syndrome. *Brain and Development* 2005, 27, 34-38.

[15] Hayashi, M; Itoh, M; Araki, S; Kumada, S; Shiod,a K; Tamagawa, K; Mizutani, T; Morimatsu, Y; Minagawa, M; Oda, M. Oxidative stress and disturbed glutamate transport in hereditary nucleotide repair disorders. *Journal of Neuropathology and Experimental Neurology* 2001, 60, 350-356.

[16] Freeman, JM. Rasmussen's syndrome: progressive autoimmune multifocal encephalopathy. *Pediatric Neurology* 2005, 32, 295-299.

[17] Rogers, SW; Andrews, PI; Gahring, LC; Whisenand, T; Cauley, K; Crain, B; Hughes, TE; Heinemann, SF; McNamara, JO. Autoantibodies to glutamate receptor GluR3 in Rasmussen's encephalitis. *Science* 1994, 265, 648-651.

[18] Bien, CG; Granata, T; Antozzi, C; Cross, JH; Dulac, O; Kurthen, M; Lassmann, H; Mantegazza, R; Villemure, JG; Spreafico, R; Elger, CE. Pathogenesis, diagnosis and treatment of Rasmussen encephalitis. A European consensus statement. *Brain* 2005, 128, 454-471.

[19] Takahashi, Y; Mori, H; Mishima, M; Watanabe, M; Fujiwara, T; Shimomura J; Aiba, H; Miyajima, T; Saito, Y; Nezu, A; Nishida, H; Imai, K; Sakaguchi, N; Kondo, N. Autoantibodies to NMDA receptor in patients with chronic forms of epilepsia partialis continua. *Neurology* 2003, 61, 891-896.

[20] Kimura, A; Sakurai, T; Suzuki, Y; Hayashi, Y; Hozumi, I; Watanabe, O; Arimura, K; Takahashi, Y; Inuzuka, T. Autoantibodies against glutamate receptor ε2-subunit detected in a subgroup of patients with reversible

autoimmune limbic encephalitis. *European Neurology* 2007, 58, 152-158.
[21] Sakuma, H; Awaya, Y; Shiomi, M; Yamanouchi, H; Takahashi, Y; Saito, Y; Sugai, K; Sasaki, M. Acute encephalitis with refractory, repetitive partial seizures (AERRPS): a peculiar form of childhood encephalitis. *Acta Neurologica Scandinavia* 2010, 121, 251-256.
[22] Kawashima, H; Suzuki, K; Yamanaka, G; Kashiwagi, Y; Takekuma, K; Amaha, M; Takahashi, Y. Anti-glutamate receptor antibodies in pediatric enteroviral encephalitis. *International Journal of Neuroscience* 2010, 120, 99-103.
[23] Tang, Y; Shimizu, E; Dube, GR; Rampon, C; Kerchner, GA; Zhuo, M; Liu, G; Tsien, JZ. Genetic enhancement of learning and memory in mice. *Nature* 1999, 401, 63-69.
[24] Dalmau, J; Tuzun, E; Wu, HY; Masjuan, J; Rossi, JE; Voloschin, A; Baehring, JM; Shimazaki, JM; Koide, R; King, D; Mason, W; Sansing, LH; Dichter, MA; Rosenfeld, MR; Lynch, DR. Paraneoplastic anti-N-methyl-D-aspartate receptor encephalitis associated with ovarian teratomas. *Annals of Neurology* 2007, 61, 25-36.
[25] Dalmau, J; Gleichman, AJ; Hughes, EG; Rossi, JE; Peng, X; Lai, M; Dessain, SK; Rosenfeld, MR; Balice-Gordon, R; Lynch, DR. Anti-NMDA-receptor encephalitis: case series and analysis of the effects of antibodies. *Lancet Neurology* 2008, 7, 1091-1098.
[26] Pillai, SC; Gill, D; Webster, R; Howman-Giles, R; Dale, RC. Cortical hypometabolism demonstrated by PET in relapsing NMDA receptor encephalitis. *Pediatric Neurology* 2010, 43, 217-220.
[27] Gutman, GA; Chandy, KG; Grissmer, S; International Union of Pharmacology. LIII. Nomenclature and molecular relationships of voltage-gated potassium channels. *Pharmacological Review* 2005, 57, 473-508.
[28] McKnight, K; Jiang, Y; Hart, Y; Serum antibodies in epilepsy and seizure-associated disorders. *Neurology* 2005, 65, 1730-1736.
[29] Vincent, A; Buckley, C; Schott, JM; Potassium channel antibody-associtaed encephalopathy: a potentially immunotherapy-responsive form of limbic encephalitis. *Brain* 2004, 127, 701-712.
[30] Solimena, M; Folli, F; Aparisi, R; Poza, G; De Camilli, P. Autoantibodies to GABA-ergic neurons and pancreatic beta cells in stiff-man syndrome. *New England Journal of Medicine* 1990, 322, 1555-1560.

[31] Honnorat, J; Saiz, A; Giometto, B; Vincent, A; Brieva, L; de Andres, C; Maestre, J; Fabien, N; Vighetto, A; Casamitjana, R; Thivolet, C; Tavalato, B, Antoine, J; Trouillas, P; Graus, F. Cerebellar ataxia with anti-glutamic acid decarboxylase antibodies: study of 14 patients. *Archives of Neurology* 2001, 58, 225-230.

[32] Mata, S; Muscas, GC; Naldi, I; Rosati, E; Paladini, S; Cruciatti, B; Bisulli, F; Paganini, M; Mazzi, G; Sorbi, S; Tinuper, P. Non-neoplastic limbic encephalitis associated with anti-glutamic acid decarboxylase antibodies. *Journal of Neuroimmunology* 2008, 13, 155-159.

[33] Liimatainen, S; Peltola, M; Sabater, L; Fallah, M; Kharazmi, E; Haapala, AM; Dastidar, P; Knip, M; Saiz, A; Peltpla, J. Clinical significance of glutamic acid decarboxylase antibodies in patients with epilepsy. *Epilepsia* 2010, 51, 760-767.

[34] Haberlandt, E; Bast, T; Ebner, A; Holthausen, H; Klugger, G; Kravljanac, R; Kroll-Seger, J; Kurlemann, G; Makowski, C; Rostasy, K; Tuschen-Hofstatter, E; Weber, G; Vincent, A; Bien, CG. Limbic encephalitis in children and adolescents. *Archives of Disease in Children* 2011, 96, 186-191.

[35] Nano, R; Balegno, S; Vaccarone, R; Corato, M; Ceroni, M. Detection of paraneoplastic anti-neuronal-specific antibodies: comparison of different immunohistochemical techniques. *Anticancer Research* 2003, 23, 2377-2381.

[36] Swedo, SE; Leonard, HL; Garvey, M; Mittleman, B; Allen, AJ, Perlmutter, S; Lougee, L; Dow, S; Zamkoff, J; Dubbert, BK. Pediatric autoimmune neuropsychiatric disorders associated with streptococcal infections: clinical description of the first 50 cases. *American Journal of Psychiatry* 1998, 155, 264-271.

[37] Dale, RC; Church, AJ; Cardoso, F; Goddard, E; Cox, TC; Chong, WK; Williams, A; Klein, NJ; Neville, BG; Thompson, EJ; Giovannoni, G. Poststreptococcal acute disseminated encephalomyelitis with basal ganglia involvement and auto-reactive antibasal ganglia antibodies. *Annals of Neurology* 2001, 50, 588-595.

[38] Edwards, MJ; Trikouli, E; Martino, D; Bozi, M; Dale, RC; Church, AJ; Schrag, A; Lees, AJ; Quinn, NP; Giovannoni, G; Bhatia, KP. Anti-basal ganglia antibodies in patients with atypical dystonia and tics. A prospective study. *Neurology* 2004, 63, 156-158.

[39] Dale, RC; Candler, PM; Church, AJ; Wait, R; Pocock, JM; Giovannoni, G. Neuronal surface glycolytic enzymes are autoantigen targets in post-

streptococcal autoimmune CNS disease. *Journal of Neuroimmunology* 2006, 172, 187-197.

[40] Sekigawa, M; Okumura, A; Niijima, S; Hayashi, M; Tanaka, K; Shimizu, T. Autoimmune focal encephalitis shows marked hypermetabolism on positron emission tomography. *Journal of Pediatrics* 2010, 156, 158-160.

[41] Okumura, A; Kidokoro, H; Itomi, K; Maruyama, K; Kubota, T; Kondo, Y; Itomi, S; Uemura, N; Natsume, J; Watanabe, K; Morishima, T. *Pediatric Neurology* 2008, 38, 111-117.

In: Pathology: New Research
Editors: J. M. Vultagione et al.

ISBN: 978-1-62100-698-5
© 2012 Nova Science Publishers, Inc.

Chapter 5

HISTOPATHOLOGICAL INVESTIGATION IN FORENSIC AUTOPSIES

Tanuj Kanchan[1], Flora D. Lobo[2], Ritesh G. Menezes[3] and B. Suresh Kumar Shetty[1]*

[1]Department of Forensic Medicine, Kasturba Medical College, Mangalore (affiliated to Manipal University) India
[2]Department of Pathology, Kasturba Medical College, Mangalore (affiliated to Manipal University) India
[3]Department of Forensic Medicine, Srinivas Institute of Medical Sciences and Research Centre, Mangalore, India

ABSTRACT

Forensic autopsies are primarily conducted to determine the cause of death and to opine if the cause of death is in accordance with the postulated manner of death. These autopsies require photography, collection of evidentiary material and identification procedures, along with chemical analysis, histopathological evaluation, and other ancillary autopsy investigations. In cases of sudden unexpected deaths wherein even though the death may have occurred from an identifiable cause, the gross autopsy findings may be obscure or non-specific thus necessitating histopathological evaluation. Histopathological evaluation is however, not very commonly done in developing countries like India and its

---

* E-mail address: tanujkanchan@yahoo.co.in, tanuj.kanchan@manipal.edu.

significance needs to be studied and emphasized in such countries. The present study was conducted in Kasturba Medical College, Mangalore, a medical institute affiliated to Manipal University in South India to highlight the importance of histopathological evaluation in medicolegal autopsies. Two hundred forensic autopsy cases were evaluated for histopathology in the associated Department of Pathology between January 2006 and September 2007. The autopsies were conducted by the Department of Forensic Medicine and the internal organs were subjected to histopathological evaluation in the Department of Pathology. Coronary atherosclerotic diseases, pneumonia and tuberculosis were the most frequent diagnoses observed in the autopsied cases. In the present case series, we have reviewed six of the unusual cases diagnosed solely by histopathological examination of the internal organs after autopsy during the aforementioned study period. The cases reviewed included a case of choriocarcinoma clinically diagnosed as septic abortion, acute leukemia manifesting as cerebral haemorrhage due to thrombocytopenia, tuberculous myocarditis presenting as sudden cardiac death, biliary cirrhosis in a chronic alcoholic, acute haemorrhagic pancreatitis as a cause of sudden death, and a case of sudden unexpected death due to malaria. The present research highlights on the decisive role of histopathological examination and the increasing trend of its usefulness in medicolegal work in recent times in developing countries like India.

Keywords: Forensic autopsy; Histopathology; Cause of death; Sudden unexpected death; Developing country

INTRODUCTION

The forensic autopsy is a medical procedure. Such autopsies with medicolegal implications are performed by forensic pathologists, primarily to determine the cause and to opine if the cause of death is in accordance with the postulated manner of death. In addition, diagnosing infectious diseases and reporting them to appropriate agencies, providing information to families about potentially inheritable diseases, helping the investigative agencies and testifying in the court of law are some of the other objectives and sequelae of conducting a forensic autopsy. The US National Association of Medical Examiners states that "the forensic pathologist shall perform histopathogical examination in cases with no gross anatomic or toxicological cause of death" [1]. These autopsies require photography, collection of evidentiary material and identification procedures, along with chemical analysis, histopathological evaluation, and other ancillary autopsy investigations. In cases of sudden unexpected deaths wherein even though the death may have occurred from an identifiable cause, the gross autopsy findings may be obscure or non-specific thus necessitating histopathological evaluation. Histopathological evaluation is, however, not very commonly done in developing countries like India and its significance needs to be studied and emphasized in these countries. A study conducted by Molina et al. shows that when the cause and manner of death are determined by gross examination at autopsy, microscopic examination will change the cause of death in < 1% of the cases and does not affect the determination of manner of death [2]. The present research highlights on the decisive role of histolopathological examination and the increasing trend of its usefulness in medicolegal work in developing countries like India.

MATERIAL AND METHODS

Two hundred forensic autopsy cases were evaluated for histopathology in the associated Department of Pathology at Kasturba Medical College, Mangalore, South India between January 2006 and September 2007. The autopsies were conducted by the Department of Forensic Medicine and the organs were subjected to microscopic evaluation in the Department of Pathology. Coronary atherosclerotic diseases, pneumonia and tuberculosis were the most frequent diagnoses observed in the autopsied cases. In the present case series, we have reviewed six of the unusual cases diagnosed solely based on histopathological examination of the organs after autopsy during the aforementioned study period. The cases reviewed included a case of choriocarcinoma clinically diagnosed as septic abortion, acute leukemia manifesting as cerebral haemorrhage due to thrombocytopenia, tuberculous myocarditis presenting as sudden cardiac death, biliary cirrhosis in a chronic alcoholic, acute haemorrhagic pancreatitis as a cause of sudden death, and a case of sudden unexpected death due to malaria. The tissue sections were fixed in 10% formalin, processed, embedded in paraffin wax and stained with haematoxylin and eosin. Special stains like Masson's trichrome, PAS, etc. were used wherever necessary.

RESULTS AND DISCUSSION

Coronary atherosclerotic diseases, pneumonia and tuberculosis were the most frequent diagnoses observed in the autopsied cases followed by chronic venous congestion of various organs and myocardial infarction. The diagnosis in these cases was made on gross examination at autopsy and histopathological or microscopic evaluation further confirmed the diagnosis. Six of the unusual cases diagnosed solely by histopathological examination of the internal organs after autopsy are herein discussed.

Case 1: A 19-year-old unmarried girl was diagnosed as a case of septicemia. She expired while on treatment in a hospital. At autopsy, on gross examination the liver, spleen and uterus showed foci of haemorrhages. On the basis of history and autopsy findings death due to septic abortion was a likely diagnosis. Very astonishingly, the histopathology proved otherwise. Sections from the liver showed tumour metastasis with large aggregates and bilaminar pattern of cytotrophoblast and syncitiotrophoblast amidst extensive haemorrhage. No chorionic villi were seen. The spleen showed only haemorrhage and infarction. The uterus showed extensive haemorrhage and occasional trophoblastic cells in the curettage material. A diagnosis of choriocarcinoma with metastasis to the liver and splenic infarction was made [3]. Choriocarcinoma is the most aggressive form of gestational trophoblastic disease (GTD). In about 40% of cases it is seen after abortion [4]. Women with low risk metastatic GTD treated aggressively with single/multiple chemotherapy do very well. Remission rate for high rate metastatic disease is 45 – 65 % [5]. In the 1st case presented here, due to lack of an early diagnosis the patient succumbed to the disease.

Case 2: A 28-year-old woman died of cerebral haemorrhage. Autopsy revealed bilateral kidneys with multiple cysts, ranging in size from 1-5 cm, obscuring the corticomedullary junction. Sections from the kidneys and other organs including uterus, fallopian tubes, ovaries and heart revealed interstitial deposits and intravascular aggregates of small to medium sized cells, with round to oval nuclei and occasional nucleoli. Thus the histological diagnosis was acute lymphocytic leukemia with infiltration to various organs.

Involvement of the kidney in acute lymphocytic leukemia (ALL) is reported in 24% of all ALL patients [6, 7]. Commonly bilateral enlargement of the kidney is seen. Development of cystic kidney in adults is rare, though a few cases have been reported in children [8].

Case 3: A 58-year-old man died a sudden unexpected death following an acute episode of chest pain. At autopsy, the papillary muscle of the left ventricle was hypertrophied and the valve cusps were thickened. The coronaries and aorta showed atheromatous plaques. A section from the left ventricular apex showed a single epithelioid granuloma in the myocardium comprising of central caseous necrotic area surrounded by epithelioid cells, lymphocytes, plasma cells and a few Langhans giant cells. A diagnosis of tuberculous granulomatous myocarditis was made. AFB stain was, however, negative [9]. Tuberculosis related sudden death due to cardiac complications is very rare. Slavin reported involvement of the heart in 10% of the tuberculosis cases [10]. Tuberculosis of myocardium occurs as miliary tuberculosis, nodular tuberculosis or tuberculous ventricular aneurysm [11].

Case 4: A 41-year-old chronic alcoholic man died suddenly due to massive haematemesis. At autopsy, the liver showed numerous greenish-yellow, firm, non-greasy nodules. Sections from the nodules showed loss of liver architecture along with regenerative nodules. Marked fibrosis and periductal onion skinning pattern was observed. Proliferating bile ductules were seen amidst fibrotic stroma and a predominant mononuclear infiltrate. Steatosis was absent. The above pattern points to a diagnosis of sclerosing cholangitis leading to secondary biliary cirrhosis with absence of alcoholic liver disease. In general deaths due to liver disease are attributed to "fatty liver" or "alcoholic liver disease". Biliary cirrhosis presenting in a chronic alcoholic is uncommon. Secondary biliary cirrhosis is more common in males. The presentation is similar to primary biliary cirrhosis with lethargy, pruritis, and skin pigmentation [12].

Case 5: A 50-year-old man was found dead in his room. He was a known alcoholic with recent past history of malaria. Medicolegal autopsy was conducted that revealed congestion of organs. Pulmonary oedema and cerebral oedema was apparent. Stomach contents had an alcoholic odour. The pancreas was oedematous and haemorrhagic with an abdominal haemorrhage in the retro-peritoneal space. Toxicological analysis of postmortem blood sample was positive for alcohol of an unremarkable amount. Histopathology sections from the pancreas showed patchy areas of haemorrhage, inflammatory infiltrate and infarction with intervening normal pancreatic acini. Focal areas of ductular dilatation with necrosis of the ducts and surrounding interstitium were seen. Lungs showed features of shock lung [13]. Sudden death due to acute haemorrhagic pancreatitis is distinctive due to its nonspecific symptoms preceding the fatal event. The suddenness of the attack and rapidity of termination of life, without the slightest clinical manifestation remains to be emphasised [14].

Case 6: An unknown elderly man was found lying dead near the railway station in the early morning hours. The body was subjected to a medico-legal autopsy. External examination was unremarkable. Internally, the lungs and brain were oedematous. The liver was congested and the spleen was enlarged. The other organs were unremarkable on gross examination. Microscopic examination of the brain, spleen, liver, lungs, heart and kidneys revealed evidence of parasitized red blood cells with malarial pigment. Routine postmortem toxicological analysis was negative for the common illicit or prescribed drugs or pesticides [15]. Malaria should be suspected as a cause of sudden unexpected death in malaria-endemic regions and in the context of travel to such endemic regions [16].

The cases reported here are unusual in the manner of presentation or in the diseases themselves. Careful sectioning of the organs may answer many of the questions which may be perplexing to the clinician. The study of autopsy cases has many advantages. It not only helps in elucidating accurately the cause of death, thereby providing information regarding the manner of death. It also helps the pathologist, who in the process of studying the organs, encounters numerous varied pathologies which would not have been encountered in routine reporting, thus helping a pathologist academically.

The primary role of the pathologist, in examination of autopsy cases is to determine cause and manner of death. This study has shown that in the majority of cases, cause and manner of death are determined during gross examination itself, but in a few cases histopathological evaluation or microscopic examination is essential to conclude the pathologies present in relation to the cause of death. This study also shows that in cases where cause and manner of death are readily apparent at the time of autopsy, microscopic examination does add information regarding communicable and neoplastic disease processes. The present case series highlights the crucial role of histolopathological examination which benefits autopsy work. If there is a slightest doubt in the mind of a forensic pathologist as to the cause of death, there should be no hesitation on his/her part to evaluate the tissues under the microscope. Thus the unpredictable pattern of clinical diseases and the challenges faced at autopsy are made easy for final diagnosis by the diagnostic pathologist.

In developing countries like India, not much importance is paid to the ancillary autopsy investigations due to lack of appropriate facilities and lack of substantial funds allocated to the investigation of death in a scientific manner. Importance of histopathological evaluation in autopsy cases needs to be emphasized wherever necessary even in developing countries like India.

REFERENCES

[1] Christiansen LR, Collins KA. Natural death in forensic setting: a study and approach to the autopsy. *American Journal of Forensic Medicine and Pathology* 2007;28:20–23.

[2] Molina DK, Wood LE, Frost RE. Is routine histopathologic examination beneficial in all medicolegal autopsies? *American Journal of Forensic Medicine and Pathology* 2007;28:1–3.

[3] Shetty BSK, Lobo F, Harindar, Shetty M et al. Post-mortem diagnosis of gestation choriocarcinoma – A case report. *Journal of Indian Academy of Forensic Medicine* 2007; 29: 59–61.

[4] Crum CP: The female genital tarct. In: Vinay Kumar, Abul K. Abbas, Nelson Fausto: Robbins and Cotran *Pathologic Basis of Disease*, 7th ed. Philadelphia: Elsevier, 2004:1113.

[5] Cunningham FG, Leveno KJ, Bloom SL, Hauth JC, Gilstrap III LC, Wenstrom KD. *Gestational Trophoblastic Diseases*. In: Williams Obstetrics. 22nd ed. USA: McGraw Hill, 2005:282.

[6] Hann IM, Lees PD, Palmer MK, Gupta S, Morris-Jones PH. Renal size as prognostic factor in childhood acute lymphoblastic leukemia. *Cancer* 1981;48:207–209.

[7] Basker M, Scott JX, Ross B, Kirubakaran C. Renal enlargement as primary presentation of acute lymphoblastic leukemia. *Indian Journal of Cancer* 2002;39:154–156.

[8] Gupta S, Kaene S. Renal enlargement as a primary presentation of acute lymphoblastic leukemia. *British Journal of Radiology* 1985;58:893–895.

[9] Kanchan T, Nagesh KR, Lobo FD, Menezes RG. Tubercular granuloma in the myocardium *Singapore Medical Journal* 2010;51:e15–7.

[10] Slavin RE: Late generalized tuberculosis: A clinical and pathologic analysis of a diagnostic puzzle and a changing pattern. In: Sommers SC, Rosen PP (eds): *Pathology Annual*, 1981: 1. East Norwalk, Conn, Appelton-Century-Crofts, 1981:81–99.

[11] Rose AG. Cardiac tuberculosis: a study of 19 patients. *Archives of Pathology and Laboratory Medicne* 1987;111:422–426.

[12] Washington K. Inflammatory and Infectious Diseases of the Liver. In: Christine AI, Elizabeth AM: *Gastrointestinal and Liver Pathology*. Philadelphia: Elsevier, 2006:563.

[13] Shetty BSK, Boloor A, Menezes RG, Shetty M, Menon A, Nagesh KR, Pai MR, Mathai AM, Rastogi P, KanchanT, Naik R, Salian RR, Jain V,

George AT. Postmortem diagnosis of acute haemorrhagic pancreatitis. *Journal of Forensic and Legal Medicine* 2010;17:316–320.

[14] Kanchan T, Shetty M, Nagesh KR, Khadilkar U, Shetty BSK, Menon A, Menezes RG, Rastogi P, Acute haemorrhagic pancreatitis – a case of sudden death. *Journal of Forensic and Legal Medicine* 2009;16:101–103.

[15] Menezes RG, Kanchan T, Rai S, Rao PP, Naik R, Shetty BSK, Lobo SW, Chauhan A, Shetty M, Mathai AM. An autopsy case of sudden unexplained death caused by malaria. *Journal of Forensic Sciences* 2010;55:835–838.

[16] Menezes RG, Pant S, Kanchan T, Senthilkumaran S, Kharosah MA, Naik R, Babu YPR, Rao PPJ, Fazil A. Malaria: An infection with global impact. In: Peterson AM, Calamandrei GE (eds): Malaria- Etiology, Pathogenesis and Treatments. New York: Nova Science Publishers, Inc, 2011 (in press).

INDEX

A

access, 42, 51, 68
accessibility, 67
accounting, 57
acid, vii, 4, 5, 6, 7, 8, 11, 12, 13, 18, 20, 21, 22, 23, 24, 25, 26, 27, 29, 31, 32, 78
action potential, 80
acute leukemia, x, 92, 93
acute lymphoblastic leukemia, 97
acute renal failure, 77
adaptation, vii
adjustment, 61, 64
adolescents, 58, 80, 88
adults, 71, 72, 74, 94
age, vii, viii, 1, 2, 3, 7, 8, 9, 10, 11, 12, 16, 20, 41, 55, 57, 60, 63, 66, 76, 78, 83, 84
agencies, 40, 42, 92
alcohol abuse, 64, 66
alcoholic liver disease, 95
alcoholism, 66
algorithm, 31
alternative energy, 4
amino, 15, 27, 31, 77, 79
amino acid, 15, 27, 31, 77, 79
aneurysm, 46, 95
anoxia, 46
antibody, 87
antioxidant, 78
anxiety, 61, 64
aorta, 95

apex, 95
apoptosis, 78
arrest, 75
arrhythmia, 8, 13
artery, 45
aspartate, 79, 87
assessment, 39, 41, 62
astrocytes, 78
asymptomatic, 19
ataxia, 80, 83, 88
atheists, 66
atherosclerosis, 45, 46
atrophy, 84
authority, vii, 41
autoantibodies, ix, 74, 79, 80, 81, 83, 84, 86, 87
autoantigens, 80, 81
autoimmunity, 80
autonomy, 40
autopsy, vii, viii, ix, 1, 2, 3, 13, 15, 16, 20, 22, 28, 30, 35, 36, 39, 40, 42, 43, 44, 45, 46, 47, 48, 49, 50, 51, 52, 53, 55, 58, 59, 60, 61, 65, 67, 68, 69, 70, 71, 72, 75, 76, 77, 78, 85, 91, 92, 93, 94, 95, 96, 97, 98
autosomal recessive, 16, 20
aversion, 66
awareness, 68

B

basal ganglia, ix, 74, 81, 83, 84, 88

beef, 27
behavioral disorders, 11
behaviors, 61, 67, 83
benefits, 48, 96
bias, 68
bile, 16, 27, 95
bile duct, 95
biliary cirrhosis, x, 92, 93, 95
bleeding, 46, 76, 77
blends, 40
blood, 12, 14, 15, 16, 18, 22, 27, 28, 30, 31, 48, 75, 95
bonds, 7
brain, ix, 4, 8, 50, 73, 75, 76, 77, 78, 81, 83, 84, 85, 86, 96
brainstem, 75, 76, 77, 78
breathing, 2
bronchiolitis, 76

C

campaigns, 3, 39
cancer, 81
candidates, 20, 39
carbon, 4, 5
cardiac arrest, 45
cardiac arrhythmia, 7
cardiac tamponade, 45
cardiomyopathy, 7, 8, 9, 10, 11, 12, 23
cation, 4, 6, 22
cell membranes, 20
cerebellum, 81
cerebral contusion, 44
cerebral cortex, ix, 74, 76, 77, 78, 81, 83
cerebral hemisphere, 76
cerebrospinal fluid, 78
cerebrum, 75, 76
certificate, 36, 45, 46, 48
challenges, 42, 96
chemical, ix, 91, 92
chemotherapy, 94
child abuse, vii, 1, 2
childhood, ix, 9, 10, 21, 27, 73, 79, 85, 87, 97

children, vii, ix, 7, 21, 27, 32, 64, 73, 74, 75, 79, 80, 81, 83, 84, 88, 94
cholangitis, 95
chorea, 81, 83, 84
choriocarcinoma, x, 92, 93, 94, 97
chorionic villi, 94
chromatography, 13
chromosome, 16, 17, 18
cirrhosis, 95
civil society, 39
classification, 2, 21
cleavage, 5
clinical application, 13
clinical diagnosis, 13, 71
clinical presentation, 25
clinical symptoms, 17, 52
coding, 62, 68
codon, 17
coenzyme, 24, 25, 26, 28, 32, 33
cognition, 65
collagen, 74
color, iv
coma, 7, 8, 10, 18
communication, 42
communities, 67
community, viii, 48, 55, 56, 57, 58, 60, 66, 67, 68
competing interests, 69
complications, 10, 32, 95
computed tomography, 76, 82, 84
computer, 31
congenital adrenal hyperplasia, 19
consciousness, 13, 83, 84
consensus, 36, 47, 53, 62, 68, 86
controversial, 17, 20, 45
convergence, 41
convulsion, 10
coronary artery disease, 45
correlation, 24
cortex, 76, 77, 78, 83
cost, 45, 67
crown, 37
cytoplasm, 84

Index

D

data set, 51, 52
deaths, ix, 2, 21, 36, 37, 38, 39, 44, 45, 46, 48, 49, 50, 51, 52, 58, 91, 93, 95
defects, 3, 29
deficiencies, 9, 14, 16, 19, 23, 29
deficiency, 5, 7, 8, 9, 10, 11, 12, 13, 14, 15, 16, 17, 18, 19, 22, 23, 24, 25, 26, 27, 28, 29, 30, 31, 32, 33
degradation, 4, 17
dehydration, 10
delusions, 66
demographic data, 63
deposition, 75
deposits, 75, 94
depression, 61, 65
depressive symptoms, 66, 71
detachment, 41
detectable, 27
detection, 18, 19, 20, 38, 51, 79, 81
developed countries, 3, 58, 66, 67
developing countries, viii, x, 55, 56, 58, 72, 91, 93, 96
diagnostic markers, 30
diarrhea, 75
dilated cardiomyopathy, 11
diseases, vii, x, 3, 14, 19, 20, 28, 32, 51, 74, 92, 93, 94, 96
disorder, 5, 7, 16, 24, 25, 26, 50, 59, 64, 65, 79
disseminated intravascular coagulation, 75
distress, 2, 50
distribution, 63
doctors, viii, 39, 48, 51, 55, 57, 60
dominance, viii, 35, 39
double bonds, 7
drugs, 96
dystonia, 81, 83, 88

E

edema, 75, 76, 77, 78
education, 47, 63, 67
electron, 6
electrons, 5, 12
emission, 82, 84
emotional distress, 60
encephalitis, vii, ix, 73, 74, 75, 76, 77, 78, 79, 80, 81, 83, 84, 85, 86, 87, 88, 89
encephalomyelitis, 82, 83, 88
encephalopathy, vii, ix, 10, 11, 17, 25, 29, 73, 74, 75, 76, 77, 78, 79, 81, 83, 84, 85, 86, 87
endothelium, 20
energy, 4, 61
energy supply, 4
enlargement, 94, 97
enterovirus, 79
enzyme, 5, 7, 8, 9, 10, 11, 12, 17, 24, 25, 29, 78, 81, 88
epidemic, 85
epidemiology, 22, 25, 70
epilepsy, 11, 64, 76, 80, 85, 87, 88
epistemology, 40
ester, 4
ethylene, 2
ethylene glycol, 2
etiology, 79
evidence, viii, 35, 38, 39, 41, 43, 45, 49, 50, 53, 71, 79, 96
examinations, viii, ix, 2, 3, 47, 50, 73, 74
excitotoxicity, 78
exclusion, 53
excretion, 12, 18, 25
exercise, 45
exons, 16, 17, 18
expertise, 40, 41, 42, 53

F

fallopian tubes, 94
fasting, 4, 5, 8, 10, 11, 18
fat, 75
fatty acids, 4, 7, 9, 25
fetus, 20
fever, 75, 77
fibroblasts, 18, 21, 23
fibrosis, 95

financial, 38, 61, 63, 64, 67
force, 38
formaldehyde, 18
formation, 5, 29
fractures, 44
free radicals, 20
functional analysis, 28
funds, 96

G

general practitioner, 69
genes, 8, 17
genetic disease, 27
genetic disorders, 30
genotype, 24, 26, 29
gestation, 97
glial cells, 78, 81, 83
globus, 83
glucose, 18, 82
glutamate, ix, 74, 79, 86, 87
glutamic acid, ix, 74, 80, 88
glycogen, 4, 13
governance, 40
government policy, 40
granules, 13
growth, 9
guidance, 40, 47

H

hallucinations, 66
haplotypes, 28
head injuries, 44, 45
health, ix, 32, 56, 57, 58, 61, 63, 64, 67, 69, 70, 72
heart disease, 48
hegemony, 37
height, 57, 63
hemiparesis, 79
hepatocytes, 13
hepatomegaly, 7, 8, 9, 10
heterozygote, 16
hippocampus, ix, 74, 78, 81, 84

histochemistry, 75
history, vii, viii, 1, 3, 35, 39, 41, 48, 61, 63, 64, 66, 94, 95
homes, 60
homicide, 37, 49, 50
hospital death, 53
human, 5, 9, 22, 24, 25, 26, 30, 42, 81
hyperinsulinism, 11
hypertension, 13
hypoglycemia, 8, 9, 10, 11, 12, 13, 22
hypothesis, 71
hypothyroidism, 19

I

identification, ix, 23, 24, 27, 29, 91, 92
identity, 36, 37, 60
ideology, 41
image, 68
immunoglobulin, 81, 82, 83
immunohistochemistry, 29, 78, 81, 82, 83
immunoreactivity, ix, 74, 75, 81, 83, 84
immunotherapy, 79, 87
improvements, 51, 74
incidence, ix, 18, 74, 81
income, 56
individuals, 60, 61, 62, 64, 65, 66, 67
industries, 56
infancy, vii, viii, 1, 2, 3, 7, 10, 14, 21, 28, 76, 85
infants, viii, 2, 3, 8, 13, 21, 22, 30
infarction, 45, 94, 95
infection, vii, 1, 2, 3, 10, 76, 80, 83, 85, 98
inflammation, vii
inflammatory mediators, 20
influenza, vii, ix, 73, 74, 75, 76, 77, 78, 85, 86
influenza a, 85
influenza virus, vii, ix, 73, 74, 75, 76, 77, 78
informed consent, 60
inhibition, 19
injuries, 44, 45, 50
institutions, viii, 2, 3, 36
instrumental support, 66
insulin, 26

Index

integration, 59
interrelations, 71
intervention, 19, 39, 67
ionization, 19, 31
irritability, 7
ischaemic heart disease, 45, 46
islands, 56
isolation, 59
isoleucine, 5
issues, 47

J

jumping, 57, 63
juries, 38
jurisdiction, 38, 51, 53
justification, 43, 48, 51

K

kidney, 23, 94
kidneys, 94, 96

L

lactic acid, 77
law enforcement, 42
laws, 40
lead, 18, 20, 49, 51, 74
learning, 79, 87
left ventricle, 95
legislation, 38, 44, 50
lesions, 77, 78, 85, 86
lethargy, 7, 10, 95
leukemia, 94
level of education, 66
liberalism, 40
lifetime, 61, 64
limbic system, 81
linoleic acid, 12
lipid peroxidation, 78
lipolysis, 4
liquid chromatography, 13

liver, 7, 8, 10, 12, 13, 14, 18, 19, 20, 24, 27, 32, 33, 75, 76, 77, 94, 95, 96
low risk, 94
lying, 96
lymphocytes, 95

M

magnetic resonance, 76, 82
major depression, 59
majority, 45, 46, 51, 67, 96
malaise, 10
malaria, x, 92, 93, 95, 96, 98
man, 40, 87, 94, 95, 96
management, 32, 40, 67
manganese, 77, 78
marital status, 61
mass, 13, 21, 25, 30, 31, 32
mass spectrometry, 13, 21, 25, 30, 31, 32
materials, 68
matrix, 4, 5, 7
matter, 77
median, 65, 80
mediastinum, 76
medical, viii, x, 22, 31, 35, 36, 37, 38, 39, 41, 42, 43, 44, 46, 47, 48, 51, 52, 53, 64, 74, 92
medication, 41, 61, 64, 78
medicine, 37, 38, 39, 40, 42
memory, 79, 87
meningitis, 74
messages, 50
metabolism, 5, 7, 25, 27, 30, 31, 32
metabolites, 12
metabolized, 4
metastasis, 94
metastatic disease, 94
methodology, 19, 58, 68
methylmalonic acidemia, 2
methylprednisolone, 82, 83, 84
mice, 87
microscope, 96
migration, 61
miliary tuberculosis, 95
mitochondria, 4, 24

models, 71
modernity, 37, 40, 41
molecular weight, 84
molecules, 79
mood disorder, 64
morphological abnormalities, viii, 2, 3
mortality, ix, 9, 38, 48, 56, 58, 73, 74, 75
mortality rate, 9, 56
multiple persons, 64
multiple regression, 66
murder, 2, 20, 50
muscles, 7
mutation, 7, 8, 9, 11, 14, 16, 17, 18, 22, 24, 27, 28, 29, 30
myalgia, 8
myocardial infarction, 45, 46, 48, 94
myocarditis, x, 92, 93, 95
myocardium, 95, 97
myopathy, 11, 13, 26, 77

N

narratives, 41
necrosis, vii, 75, 76, 77, 85, 95
neuroblastoma, 80
neurons, 76, 77, 78, 81, 83, 84, 87
neuropathy, 13
nodules, 95
normal development, 75
nuclei, 78, 94
nucleus, 75
nurses, 65

O

objectivity, 41
occlusion, 45
oedema, 95
organ, 8, 18, 20, 39, 41, 75, 92, 93, 94, 95, 96
ovaries, 94
overlap, 11
oxidation, vii, 4, 5, 6, 7, 8, 10, 11, 12, 13, 20, 21, 22, 23, 24, 25, 26, 27, 29, 32

oxidative stress, ix, 74, 78, 86

P

pain, 9, 56, 94
pancreas, 95
pancreatitis, x, 92, 93, 95, 98
parallel, 38
paralysis, 83
paraneoplastic syndrome, 80
parents, 64
partial seizure, 79, 87
participants, 60, 69
pathogenesis, ix, 33, 73, 74, 78, 79, 84
pathologist, viii, 2, 3, 42, 43, 50, 52, 92, 96
pathology, vii, 38, 40, 51
pathophysiology, 20
pedagogy, 40
peripheral neuropathy, 10
peritoneum, 76
personality, 59
pharyngitis, 81
phenotype, 24, 26, 28, 29, 81
phenylalanine, 19, 30
phenylketonuria, 19, 30
phosphate, 18
physicians, 75
pigmentation, 95
pilot study, 19
placenta, 20
plasma cells, 95
plasma membrane, 4
platelets, 13, 19
pneumonia, x, 92, 93, 94
police, viii, 36, 38, 39, 44, 50, 55, 57, 58, 60, 61, 68
policy, 40
politics, 39
polymorphisms, 17, 18
polypeptide, 7, 8, 11
population, viii, 13, 18, 22, 30, 46, 55, 56, 57, 67, 70
positron, 82, 89
potassium, ix, 74, 80, 87
precedents, 39

predictive accuracy, 44
pregnancy, 13, 19, 20, 32, 33
premature death, 48
preparation, iv, 19
preparedness, 69
prevention, ix, 51, 56, 57, 59, 67, 68, 70, 72, 79
primary biliary cirrhosis, 95
primary function, 51
prisons, 36
problem-solving, ix, 56
professionals, 36, 57, 67
prognosis, 74, 83
prophylaxis, ix, 73, 74
psychiatric diagnosis, 61, 62, 63, 64, 65, 68, 69
psychiatric disorders, 59, 64, 65
psychiatric illness, 59
psychological problems, 61
psychology, 40
psychopathology, vii, viii, 55
psychosocial factors, 62, 63, 64
public concern, 57
public education, 67
public health, 19, 51, 56, 58
public interest, 38
public resources, 40
publishing, 51
pulmonary edema, 9
pulmonary embolism, 45
punishment, 58

Q

qualifications, 38, 41
qualitative research, 68

R

reactions, 5, 58, 78
reading, 50
reasoning, 51
recall, 68
recession, 59

recognition, ix, 56, 67, 75
recommendations, 51
red blood cells, 96
registries, 48
regression, 59, 62, 66
regression analysis, 62, 66
regression model, 59, 62
regulations, 40
relatives, 58, 60, 61, 64, 65
religion, 58, 66, 71
repair, 86
researchers, 44
reserves, 4
resources, 46
respiratory acidosis, 12
response, 4, 27, 43
responsiveness, 7, 79
retinopathy, 10
revenue, 37
rhabdomyolysis, 7, 9, 10, 11, 12, 13
rights, 41
risk, viii, 3, 14, 32, 43, 48, 51, 55, 56, 59, 65, 66, 67, 68, 70, 71, 72
rules, 42

S

safety, 51
saturated fat, 7
scavengers, 78
schizophrenia, 61, 64, 66, 71
school, 61
science, vii, 1, 2, 3, 37, 41, 42
scientific investigations, 39
scientific method, 42
secretion, 26
seizure, 87
sensitivity, 68
sequencing, 16
serum, ix, 74, 79, 83, 84
sex, viii, 55, 60
shock, 46, 75, 76, 77, 85, 95
signs, 11
skeletal muscle, 11
skin, 95

society, 40, 41, 56, 66
solution, 18, 68
specialists, 69
species, 5, 12
spleen, 94, 96
splenic infarction, 94
stabilization, 29
state, 5, 39, 40, 41, 52
state intervention, 40
states, 43, 92
statistics, 48
status epilepticus, 76
steroids, 81
storage, 11, 26
stress, 41, 71, 78, 86
stressors, 65
stroke, 77, 86
stroma, 95
subacute, ix, 74, 81, 84
substance abuse, 64
substitution, 17
substitutions, 17, 18
substrate, 5, 11
substrates, 5
sudden infant death syndrome, vii, viii, 1, 2, 21, 25, 27, 28
suicidal behavior, 59, 71
suicide, vii, viii, 37, 41, 44, 45, 50, 55, 56, 57, 58, 59, 60, 62, 63, 64, 65, 66, 67, 68, 69, 70, 71, 72
supplementation, 18
survival, 68
survivors, 72
susceptibility, 30
swelling, 76
symptoms, 7, 11, 12, 23, 79, 80, 84, 95
syndrome, vii, 1, 8, 12, 13, 19, 21, 33, 75, 76, 77, 78, 80, 85, 86, 87

T

target, 40, 58
techniques, 88
tension, viii, 35, 37
testing, 19

thalamus, ix, 74, 75, 76, 77, 78, 83
therapy, 12, 18, 83
thrombocytopenia, x, 92, 93
thrombus, 46
tics, 81, 88
tissue, ix, 8, 44, 46, 52, 73, 93
toxicology, 50
traditions, 53
translation, 61
transport, 22, 86
transportation, 4
trauma, 44
treatment, ix, 48, 56, 61, 63, 64, 67, 78, 79, 82, 83, 84, 86, 94
tremor, 83
trial, 50, 78
tuberculosis, x, 92, 93, 94, 95, 97
tumors, 80
tyrosine, 19, 30

U

universe, 66
upper respiratory infection, 16
upper respiratory tract, 10
urine, 12, 19, 25, 28, 30
uterus, 94

V

vaccinations, ix, 73, 74
validation, 19
valve, 95
variables, 62, 63
variations, 28
vessels, 75, 77, 78
victims, viii, 50, 55, 57, 58, 60, 63, 64
viral infection, 85
viscera, 10, 27
vision, 41
vomiting, 2, 10, 11, 13

W

weakness, 7
welfare, 40
well-being, 70
white matter, 77
witnesses, 50
worldwide, viii, 19, 55, 56, 69
wound healing, vii

X

xeroderma pigmentosum, 86

Y

yield, 5, 49
young people, 56, 69